THEORIES OF HEALTH CARE COST-EFFECTIVENESS ANALYSIS

RICHARD ERNST

outskirts
press

Outskirts Press, Inc.
http://www.outskirtspress.com

Paperback ISBN: 978-1-4787-8329-9

Outskirts Press and the "OP" logo are trademarks belonging to Outskirts Press, Inc.

PRINTED IN THE UNITED STATES OF AMERICA

Contents

Theories of Health Care Cost-Effectiveness Analysis

Theories of Health Care Cost-Effectiveness Analysis

1 Introduction to Health Care Cost-Effectiveness Analysis

1.1 The Background

The essence of health care cost-effectiveness analysis (CEA) is a set of decision rules the use of which enables public health care agencies to choose the most socially beneficial treatments for their patient communities. The subject matter of CEA is still new, and it has developed only slowly and somewhat irregularly over the past several decades. Nonetheless, two basic forms of CEA are now recognized. In the first form, which will be called *global CEA*, the health care agency's goal is to distribute all of its patients among treatments for their illnesses and other health problems. In the second form, here called *single-treatment CEA*, the agency's task is to decide whether or not to provide or insure one— usually new—treatment for a specific illness or other health care problem. In both forms it will be assumed here that the agency operates with a budget or health care spending limit set by some superior funding authority. When it uses CEA, the health care agency's decisions about which treatments to provide or sanction for its patients are conditional on its budget, and each time its budget is changed the set of treatments determined to be "cost-effective"—the treatments that should be provided to or insured for patients—ordinarily changes as well.

The first authors to use the term "cost-effectiveness analysis" for health care were Klarman, Francis, and Rosenthal [1968] who compared the annual costs of two treatments for chronic renal disease, hemodialysis and kidney transplantation. In their study patients' health wellbeing was defined as a year of life gained by treatment, and the treatment having the smaller of the two costs per year of life gained was said to be "cost-effective". This type of evaluation in which the health outcomes of two or more treatments for a medical problem are or are assumed to be identical and the least-cost treatment is declared cost-effective is now known as *cost-minimization analysis* and is a minor and infrequently used variant of the single-treatment form of CEA. A number of experimental attempts have been made to set out the general theory of CEA in the past half century, but only a handful of them have been recognized and accepted by practitioners. In the early 1970s Weinstein and Zeckhauser [1973] claimed that the rules for making many kinds of resource allocation decisions involve the comparison of a numerical measure of the given health care system's performance with a critical ratio. The argument has sometimes been cited as the fundamental basis of CEA, but it is only loosely applicable to the single-treatment form and it has no obvious bearing on the global form. By the late 1970s it became evident that the methods of global CEA involve the ranking of treatments by their marginal costs of producing the health care benefits (Shepard and Thompson [1979]).   However, not until the mid-1990s was it demonstrated—by means of a numerical example and without proof—how these treatment rankings enter into the rules for choosing a socially desirable distribution of patients to treatments (Karlsson and Johannesson [1996]). Only in 1999 some two decades after the existence of the rules was intuited did the first effort to prove the optimality of the rules appear (Laska et al. [1999]). And what is the most promising and useful recent addition to the theory of single-treatment CEA, the concept of net monetary or health net benefits, dates only from the late 1990s (Stinnett and Mullahy [1998]).

Therefore, much of the theoretical foundation of CEA and particularly that of the single-treatment form remains vague and unsettled. For example, It has been written variously that CEA lacks a single theoretical foundation and that its procedures are derived from several or more different sources (Garber et al. [1996], Neumann [2005]), that it is a methodology for ranking many treatments for different illnesses according to their "effectiveness" (Johannesson and Weinstein [1993]), that it is only a methodology for comparing two treatments for one illness [Neumann, 2005], and that it may or may not be merely a special form of cost-benefit analysis (Weinstein and Stason [1977], Phelps and Mushlin [1991], Pauley [1995], Drummond et al. [1997], Russell [2000]). That there are two forms of CEA is seldom mentioned by researchers and the logical connections between the two have yet to be examined. But perhaps most significantly, the ethical basis of and societal justification for single-treatment CEA have never been made clear. What sort of wellbeing the single-treatment form confers on society, why it is good to choose a "cost-effective" treatment rather than some other treatment for patients, and why the single-treatment form should be used at all in public health care policy are questions that remain little discussed and unresolved.

The record of the many hundreds of published applications of single-treatment CEA is also mixed. Although the rigor of these studies has improved over time, reviews of their quality have been decidedly critical (Udvarhelyi et al. [1992], Neumann et al. [2000], Marshall et al. [2002], Spiegel et al. [2004], Drummond and Sculpher [2005], Neumann et al. [2005]), and one can easily come away from these reviews with the impression that much of the empirical literature using CEA is untrustworthy. Most of the criticism centers on the misuse of elemental definitions and data, but the imprecision of the accepted theory of CEA almost certainly also figures into the errors made by researchers and policy authorities alike.

Single-treatment CEA is now used by government health care agencies in the United Kingdom, some of the Commonwealth nations, and at least nominally in European countries like Spain. However, with one notable exception neither form of CEA has been used by health care agencies in the US. The exception is the application of global CEA in the design of the Oregon's Medicaid Plan during the late 1980s and early 1990s, and even there the final design of the Plan only vaguely approximated the format that a rigorous application of CEA would have produced. The many reasons why US health care agencies resist CEA have become the subject of a small body of literature (e.g., Berger and Teutch [2005], Luce [2005], Neuman [2005], Siegel [2005]), and are said to range from ideological hostility to any form of health care planning to the welfare definitions of CEA and fears that measurements of the variables used in empirical CEAs are open to manipulation, bias, or error. All the same, unless the fraction of gross domestic income spent on health care in the US is allowed to grow without limit, the perception that government spending on health care must be constrained is likely to gain ground. Hence at some point a means for allocating fixed public health care budgets among the competing demands for health care—a means that CEA provides—should become increasingly appealing even to those who now oppose it.

The purpose of this book is therefore to set out and justify as completely as possible the correct decision rules of CEA in order to make them understandable to readers concerned with the design and administration of health care policy. The book draws together and in extends what is currently known about these rules, and it shows that the rules can be derived from economic models in the same way as the theorems of welfare economics are derived from models of consumer and producer behavior.

1.2 The Model Health Care Agency in Cost-Effectiveness Analysis

The central entity in CEA is a model health care agency—more commonly referred to as a "decision-maker" in the CEA literature—that serves a given community and whose function it is to provide, cause to be provided, or otherwise facilitate the provision of health care to persons in that community who have health problems. In this book the model agency is assumed to undertake this activity so as to produce health wellbeing for its community, and it is characterized by the following features:

4

• The agency is either an insurer of (a payer for) health care such as the Medicare program and Medicaid plans in the US, or a direct provider such as the UK's National Health Service.

• It serves a well-defined patient population or community having a well-defined set of illnesses and other health problems.

• It operates with a budget set and maintained by a superior funding authority. Nothing in the principles of CEA actually requires that the agency be publicly owned, but because private health care providers are likely to have organizational objectives other than or in addition to producing health wellbeing for their communities, it will be assumed that the model health care agency is publicly owned.

• If it is a provider it produces health care. If it is an insurer it directs private and other public providers to the production of health care, and it does this not by command but by a system of reimbursement and utilization rules.

• It is able to direct, channel, or guide patients to the treatments it produces or sanctions. It may do this by any one or more of a number of methods: for example, by means of the recommendations, referrals, or orders from the health professionals it employs or whom it reimburses; by its copayment structure and eligibility requirements; by the health care information it furnishes to patients; and so forth.

In this book the decision rules of CEA are derived from two models of health care agencies' behavior. The first of the two is attributable to MC Weinstein, and it will be used to deduce the rules for both global and single-treatment CEA. As has been said, theoretical structures and formulations are uncommon in the CEA literature, but early in the development of the discipline Weinstein offered a normative premise regarding agencies' goal-seeking behavior, and insofar as there exists a classical welfare foundation of CEA it is Weinstein's premise. The premise is not accepted or even recognized by all practitioners of CEA, but the conventional decision rules of CEA can be derived from the model

5

of a health care agency that behaves in a manner consistent with the this premise. In 1977 Weinstein wrote:

> "(T)he underlying premise of cost-effectiveness in health problems is that, for any given level of resources available, society (or the decision-making jurisdiction involved) wishes to maximize the total aggregate health benefits conferred..."

(Weinstein and Stason [1977]), and the same or similar statements appear elsewhere in his work (Weinstein and Fineberg [1980], Johannesson and Weinstein [1993], Garber, Weinstein, et al [1996]). That is, according to Weinstein's "underlying premise" the health care agency ("the decision-making jurisdiction") should seek to maximize its community's ("society's") total health benefits subject to constraints on the sizes of the flows of services from its stock of productive resources. As it stands the premise is not workable because it is not possible to aggregate or quantify a physical "level" of productive resources. But since a total stock or flow of productive resources can always be aggregated by its cost, it is useful to employ a slightly different but equivalent version of Weinstein's premise for deriving the decision rules of CEA.

Weinstein's Axiom: The health care agency should choose a set of treatments for health problems so that if patients are assigned to these treatments the community's total health benefits are maximized subject to whatever is the agency's budget or other total cost constraint.

Because it seeks a cost-constrained maximum of its entire community's health benefits, a health care agency that acts in conformity with Weinstein's Axiom will be called a *global maximizer* (GM). A GM agency seeks to optimize the allocation of its health care resources, and it is now well established in the CEA literature that the model health care agency in the theory of global CEA is a global maximizer. But it is, perhaps, testimony to the disconnectedness of the overall theory of CEA that Weinstein's Axiom and the GM agency model have never been used to justify the decision rules of single-illness CEA.

It seems fair to say that until recently the welfare foundation of single-treatment CEA has been regarded as self-evident and largely ignored by practitioners, but in the past decade and a half an explicit normative premise known as *willingness to pay* (WTP) has emerged in the literature and been applied to the single-treatment form. Briefly put, the WTP premise holds that a health care agency should set a maximum money amount or highest "price" it is willing to pay for an additional unit of its community's health benefits. The price is set either arbitrarily by the health care agency or according to the observed preferences of its patient community. A new treatment is then deemed acceptable for patients if its marginal cost of producing health benefits is no greater than this highest price. The WTP premise is discussed in the chapters that follow, and here it will be noted only that it is an alternative to and generally at odds with Weinstein's Axiom. In Chapter 3 it is shown that in the process of determining an optimal distribution of patients among all treatments for all illnesses and other health problems, the GM agency produces what can be construed as a highest optimal price or marginal cost of health benefits. It is always possible that, given the same total treatment cost, a GM agency and a health care agency that adopts the WTP premise will choose the same highest price of health benefits, but if that happens it is only by chance. Nothing in Weinstein's Axiom and the WTP premise force the two highest prices to be the same, and if they are not, GM and WTP agencies will not necessarily reach the same conclusions about the cost-effectiveness of new or other treatments for an illness.

The second model of health care agencies' behavior that will be used to derive the decision rules of CEA is, unlike the GM model, applicable only to the single-treatment form. The model, which is presented in Chapter 7, has not previously appeared in the CEA literature but is of a type sometimes used by operations researchers. The agency's behavior is known as *myopic optimization,* and the model health care agency that engages in it will be called a *myopic optimizer* (MO). Despite its simplicity the GM agency model is clearly restrictive. A real-world health care agency may lack the ability to distribute all of its patients among treatments for their health problems in a way that gives a total cost-constrained maximum of the community's total health benefits, and an MO agency is of this kind. Hence when it is confronted with the opportunity to provide or insure a new treatment for its patients, the MO agency may, if it judges the action to be justified, add the new treatment to its offerings. By a justified action it means that the agency can redistribute patients having a small number of other illnesses and health problems among treatments for those illnesses and problems so as to provide or insure the new treatment, increase or not reduce its community's total health benefits, and not increase its total cost. Moreover, if two or more of such redistributions of patients exist, the agency will always choose the one that gives the largest increase in total cost-constrained health benefits. In effect an MO agency acts myopically or short-sightedly by seeking to maximize its community's total health benefits within only a part of its health care system rather than the whole.

Strictly speaking, a GM health care agency is also a myopic optimizer. When given its total cost a GM agency moves from an initial optimal distribution of all patients to a new optimal distribution, it implicitly gains the largest attainable increase in total health benefits. However, a MO agency is not necessarily a global maximizer. Because it does not necessarily seek an optimal distribution of patients among all treatments, an MO agency may not begin its consideration of a new treatment with a total cost-constrained maximum of its community's total health benefits, and, even if it adopts the new treatment, the final distribution of its patients among all treatments may also not be optimal. All the same and despite the differences between GM and MO behavioral models, it is shown in Chapter 7 that for all practical purposes the decision rules they imply for single-treatment CEA are the same.

The ethical underpinnings of both agency models—and hence also those of the decision rules of CEA—are utilitarian in the sense of Bentham and JS Mill. That is, each agency's sole objective is to distribute its patients among treatments so as to increase or maximize its community's total health benefits subject to a spending constraint. Nothing is implied about the fairness of this distribution or of its other moral attributes. It has already been remarked that when a new treatment is provided to or insured for patients and it is more costly than other treatments for the same illness or health problem, the agency must preserve its total cost constraint by switching patients who have other illnesses or health problems from more expensive and more health-benefit productive treatments to less expensive and less health-benefit productive treatments. These latter patients lose health benefits, and CEA contains no mechanisms for compensating them for their losses or even calculating the appropriate amounts of compensation. In this way CEA differs from conventional cost-benefit analysis. The principles of cost-benefit analysis hold that a change in the agency's distribution of patients among treatments is acceptable if and only if it causes a *Pareto improvement* in the community's overall health wellbeing—if and only if the change makes at least one patient better off than before and, because they are or could be compensated for their losses of health wellbeing, no patients are necessarily left worse off than before. That the patients who lose health benefits by applications of CEA are never compensated for their losses, either conceptually or in fact, makes it hard to see that CEA is merely a special version of cost-benefit analysis.

It has been customary in single-treatment CEAs to carry out the evaluation of a new treatment by comparing it to only one other treatment. The conclusion of the CEA is then that one of the two treatments is cost-effective and that the cost-effective treatment should be provided to or insured for patients. It has long been known, however, that showing a new treatment to be cost-effective in comparison with only one other treatment is not—even if the demonstration is theoretically valid—usually sufficient to recommend it for patients when other treatment options are available to the agency. Obviously, the new treatment may be cost-effective when it is matched against one comparator treatment but not against others, and this is especially apt to be so when the chosen comparator treatment is a placebo.

In this book two definitions of cost-effectiveness will therefore be used. When in a two-way comparison of treatments A and B for some illness or health problem it is found by the appropriate decision rule that A rather than B should be provided to or insured for patients than treatment B, A will be said to be *cost-effective relative to B*. Hence relative cost-effectiveness should be understood as equivalent to unqualified cost-effectiveness in the standard CEA literature, and the single-treatment decision rules presented here for relative cost-effectiveness are the same as those customarily used to decide the unqualified cost-effectiveness of a new treatment. It will then be said that a treatment is *absolutely cost-effective* for a given illness if it is cost-effective relative to every other treatment for the illness. The definitions of relative and absolute cost-effectiveness will be made specific in the next few chapters, but the concept of absolute cost-effectiveness is particularly important because *treatments should be provided to or sanctioned for patients if and only if they are absolutely cost-effective*. In the GM model a treatment is absolutely cost-effective if and only if by selecting it the agency satisfies Weinstein's Axiom. In the MO model an absolutely cost-effective treatment must be proved to be cost-effective relative to every other treatment for the focal illness.

In single-treatment CEA the conventional test for the (relative) cost-effectiveness of a new treatment the primary decision variable is a ratio called an *incremental cost-effectiveness (ICE) ratio*. An ICE ratio is defined as the difference between the costs of two treatments A and B

10

divided by the difference between the health benefits the two treatments produce, and it is meaningful only if the denominator is positive. The ratio is commonly understood to be a special kind of marginal or incremental cost of health benefits. It is the added cost of producing health benefits by switching patients who have a given illness or health problem from the less less costly, less health-benefit productive treatment B to the more more costly, more health-benefit productive treatment A. The conventional (but incomplete) decision rule for cost-effectiveness then states that a new treatment A is cost-effective (relative to treatment B) for the given illness or health problem if the ICE ratio defined on the costs and health benefits of A and B is smaller than a certain value. This value has been given various names in the CEA literature—"the" threshold, key or critical value—and in the willingness-to-pay literature it is known as the highest price or maximum money amount a health care agency is willing to pay for an extra unit of health benefits. In this book it will be called the agency's and its health care system's *cutoff point*.

As single-illness CEA came to be used for evaluating the acceptability of new treatments it quickly became evident that the conclusions of the analyses could not be taken as certain. Treatment costs and health benefits might be estimated from several published or unpublished sources or even conjectured by analysts or their consultants. Thus the conclusions of single-treatment CEAs were no more reliable and trustworthy than the estimates of treatment costs and health benefits used to construct the test ICE ratios, and that understanding led first to the use of deterministic sensitivity analyses of the conclusions. In a deterministic sensitivity analysis the cutoff point and the parameters of the test ICE ratio are varied one or two at a time, and the test conclusion is said to be more reliable or robust the less sensitive it is to parameter variation. Partly because of the natural limitations of this kind of exercise and partly because of the growing use of sample data to estimate treatment costs and health benefits, a second type of sensitivity analysis known as probabilistic sensitivity analysis began to be used in the 1990s. It then became apparent that there was little point in applying probabilistic methods to CEAs *post hoc* when the CEA itself could be conducted probabilistically, and the methods were gradually put together in what is now known simply as *probabilistic cost-effectiveness analysis.*

The principle feature of probabilistic CEA is the characterization of treatment costs and health benefits as random variables having particular sample distributions and population parameters. Hence the decision variables of single-treatment CEA such as ICE ratios and the yes-or-no conclusions of the analyses themselves also become random variables having particular sample distributions and, possibly, estimable population parameters. Then and provided plausible assumptions can be made about the distributions of treatment costs and health benefits, useful probabilistic judgments can also be obtained about the true value of the CEA's decision variable and the cost-effectiveness of the new treatment.

The late 1990s brought about the introduction of a new decision variable for single-treatment CEAs called *net (physical or monetary) benefits.* The net benefit of a treatment is a simple linear function of its cost, its health benefit product, and the (fixed) cutoff point. The use of net benefits to assess relative and absolute cost-effectiveness is not a separate theory of health care agency behavior, but rather a theory of treatment-choice decision making. The appeal of the net benefits variable is twofold: it provides simpler rules for deciding relative and absolute cost-effectiveness than an ICE ratio; and when sample data are available, it or its sample mean can, unlike an ICE ratio and an ICE ratio sample mean, reasonably be assumed to be normally distributed. In turn, this normality property is useful for performing parametric statistical tests of cost-effectiveness in probabilistic CEAs. Net benefits decision making for single-treatment CEA is discussed at length in Chapter 8, and several examples of statistical tests for absolute cost-effectiveness using net benefits variables are described in Chapter 9.

1.3 Some Nomenclature and Conventions

Up to this point the words "illness", "health problem" and "treatment" have been used loosely, but hereafter "illness or other health problem" will be shortened to "illness", and it will denote any kind of ailment or other adverse health condition, including injuries, wounds, genetic conditions, and so on for which patients either do or are likely to seek care, and it may be actual or potential. "Treatment" denotes any sort of health or medical intervention—diagnostic, therapeutic, or preventive—in the illness. It may be a single medical, surgical, drug, or other procedure, or it may be bundle of these kinds of procedures. The expression *patient assignment*, or usually just assignment, denotes a distribution of patients among treatments. In general it will be assumed that there are I illnesses indexed by i in the agency's patient population and that there are J_i treatments indexed by j for each illness i. Hence in total there are $\sum_{i=1}^{I} J_i$ treatments for all illnesses.

With n_{ij} signifying the number of patients directed, referred, or otherwise channeled to treatment ij, a system-wide or *global patient assignment* is the $\sum_{i=1}^{I} J_i$ -tuple $(n_{11}, n_{12},\ldots,n_{IJ_i})$. That is, a global patient assignment—or just global assignment—specifies the number of patients receiving each of the $\sum_{i=1}^{I} J_i$ treatments the health care agency provides, offers, sanctions, or otherwise makes available to its members. When only one illness i is under consideration, the numbers of patients given the treatments for the illness will be called a *single-treatment patient assignment* or single-treatment assignment. As needed it will be denoted by J-tuple $(n_{i1}, n_{i2},\ldots, n_{iJ})$, or represented in short form by (n_i). Again notice that the verb "assign" should be understood in the sense of "is offered", "is sanctioned", or "is available to". It does not imply a direct command. Whether the assignment is global or single-treatment, it is effectuated by the health professionals employed or reimbursed by the agency, by the agency's copayment and eligibility rules, by health care information disseminated by the agency, or by patients' own actions.

In order to derive the decision rules of CEA from the two health care agency models it is convenient to define the agency's alternative of not providing, sanctioning, or offering care for a patient having a given illness. That is, the agency makes no treatment available for patients having the illness and there is no contact between patients and providers. This option will be called the *no-action treatment* for that illness, and a no-action treatment for each illness will always be included in the set of the agency's treatment alternatives. (Notice that no-action is not the same as placebo because placebo implies contact with a provider.) All other treatments in which some positive quantity of care is provided to, sanctioned for, or otherwise offered to patients will be called *active treatments*.

In the rest of the book it will be assumed that the cost of and health benefits produced by all no-action treatments are both zero. The assumption that the cost of not caring for patients is defended in the section 1.5. It might be argued, however, that not treating patients produces a negative quantity of health benefits for the health care agency. Patients forego health benefits when they are denied care, and it can be contended that these losses should be subtracted from the agency's total output of health benefits. The argument has some superficial appeal, but losses of health benefits are caused by illnesses and not by the agency's failure to treat. And there are, moreover, at least two other reasons why the argument is inapplicable to theories of CEA.

First, if losses of health benefits are to be charged against the agency, the cost saving that results from non-treatment should be credited to its total cost. The losses of health benefit and savings in treatment costs are both the results of the same policy. But these cost savings are not realizable and there is no way to enter them into the agency's actual money budget. Thus if the agency cannot realize the cost saving, it should not be charged losses of health benefits.

14

Second, if losses of health benefits are to be charged to the agency when it denies treatment, it is equally justifiable to credit the agency with any gains of health benefits by untreated patients when they recover from their illnesses. The losses and gains are each attributable to the same policy. But crediting the agency for the production of health benefits when it takes no part in the activities or conditions that create them is hardly defensible. Thus by the same token it is unreasonable to charge the agency for losses of health benefits when it takes no part in the activities or conditions that cause them.

Real-world health care agencies may, on account of legal mandates or because of social or political pressures, provide some minimum quantity of health care to patients having certain kinds of illnesses, and for these illnesses there are no no-action treatments. Techniques for incorporating minimum-care constraints into global CEA exist but there are no genuinely satisfactory ways of embodying them in single-treatment CEA. Moreover, any kind of minimum care constraint imposed on the agency or one that it creates itself is or can be in conflict with the agency's utilitarian welfare objective. By diverting its resources to the production of minimum care for some patients or groups of illnesses, the model agency cannot necessarily maximize or attain the largest possible increase in the total quantity of its community's health benefits. In this book it will consequently be assumed that the health care agency operates without constraints on the minimum costs of care that it provides to or insures for its patients.

1.4 Health Benefits in Cost-Effectiveness Analysis

The two principal components of CEAs are the costs and health benefits of treatments for illnesses. Various conceptual and empirical problems arise in the definitions and measurement of these quantities, but there are now large literatures on both health benefits and treatment costs and with a few exceptions these problems will not be discussed here. It will be assumed that the health benefits product of every treatment is a constant and that the health benefits of all active treatments are given information.

So far the term "health benefits" has been referred to as if it were self-explanatory, but it is appropriate to give operational meaning to the term. Although the health benefits of treatments are now defined generally as measurable quantities of health or health wellbeing, in the history of CEA these quantities have been defined and measured in many different ways: for example, as years of life extension due to treatment, the time to recurrence or cure of a disease, the number of correctly diagnosed tumors of a particular kind, millimeters of reduction in systolic blood pressure, changes in white blood cell count, and so on. The difficulty with most of these definitions of health benefits and especially those in which benefits are specified as medical outcomes is that they cannot be generalized across different types of diseases and other health problems. Hence they are of no use for systematic health care decision-making. For instance, there are no immediate ways of comparing the substantive health benefits defined alternatively as the reduction in the number of post-menopausal womens' hip fractures due to drug treatment for osteoporosis and changes in HDL-LDL ratios in patients who receive statin drugs. If a health care agency seeks to maintain a larger rather than smaller quantity of health wellbeing for its overall patient community yet lacks the resources to care optimally for all patients suffering from osteoporosis and atherosclerosis, it must deny the optimally effective treatment to some patients suffering from one of the two ailments. But it has no coherent means of allocating its limited resources between the two groups of patients because the number of hip fractures and changes in HDL-LDL ratios are not comparable measures of health benefits.

The problem raised by illness- or condition-specific definitions of health benefits has led researchers who use CEA, especially those in the US and the UK, to employ a generic measure of health benefits called health-related *quality-adjusted life years*, or QALYs for short. A QALY is simply a year of life weighted by a numerical measure of health status or health wellbeing known as *health-related quality of life* (QOL). The measure is scaled from 0 which is associated with the worst possible health state—typically death—to 1 which is associated with perfect health. Hence 8 months of treatment for an illness during which a patient's QOL averages 0.75 yields 0.5 QALYs for that patient and the treatment for her illness.

A large number of generic QOL measures has been proposed in the literature on CEA and in health economics generally, and many of them have been or are in use. (For a few of the many surveys of the literature see, e.g., Drummond et al. [1997], Coons et al. [2000], Mishoe and Maclean [2001], Fayers and Hays [2005], and Feeny [2005]). Broadly speaking they are of two types. One defines QOL in terms of patients' states of health. The other defines it in terms of the wellbeing patients experience from these states of health. CEAs in which QOL measures are of the latter type are often called *cost-utility analyses*. Health and wellbeing measures of health benefits are both computed from responses to questionnaires given to patients, patient surrogates, or others, and both may be of the single- or multi-attribute form. An example of a utility-related (and single-attribute) measure, is known as the time-tradeoff measure. There are variants of the measure, but in its basic form a respondent is asked to decide how many months or years $Y_{healthy}$ of a remaining lifetime in perfect health she would give up in order to avoid spending a given number or months or years Y_{ill} ($\leq Y_{healthy}$) in a particular state of ill health. The measure can then be defined as $Y_{ill}/Y_{healthy}$, and it varies between 1, when the experience of ill health is no different from the experience of perfect health, and 0 for death. Examples of (multi-attribute) health-related measures are those obtained from the Rand Short-Form 36-Item (SF-36) questionnaire, perhaps the most widely used of all QOL survey instruments. The SF-36 employs a set of weights to reduce subjects' numerical responses to 36 questions to eight "domain" or dimension values representing an individual's state of health. Each of the eight domain values can be rescaled to a number from 0 to 1 and employed as a measure of QOL. There appear to be no compelling methodological reasons for choosing between utility- and health-related QOL measures for CEAs, and the selection can be left to the health care agency's or analyst's taste or made on account of practical considerations such as the costs of gathering the data necessary for estimating them.

The claim or assumption that utility-related QOL-related measures represent utility as economists understand the word does, however, raise problems. For more than a century it has been a tenet of economic theory that utility is not numerically measurable, and apparently on that account the authors of tracts on CEA (e.g., Drummond et al. [1997], O'Connor [2004], Coons and Shaw [2005]) have begun to replace the word "utility" in utility-related measures of health benefits with the word "preferences". By this rewording $QOL_1 > QOL_2$ implies only that experiencing health state 1 is preferred to experiencing health state 2, and it is not to be taken that either the difference $QOL_1 - QOL_2$ or the ratio QOL_1/QOL_2 is numerically meaningful. Since QALYs in particular and health benefits in general are the products of QOL and time experiencing QOLs, it is likewise the case that they order states of health wellbeing, but that differences in or ratios of QALYs and other measures of health benefits are also not numerically meaningful. Various tests for the validity and reliability of QOL measures have been developed by researchers during the past two decades (see, e.g., Dijkers [1999], Bowling [2001], Mishoe and Maclean [2001], O'Connor [2004], or Hays and Revicki [2005]), but it can always be argued that all numerical measurements of health states and health state preferences are ultimately subjective, and therefore that the ordering of any measure of health benefits is disputable. In one sense the criticism is only a quibble inasmuch as many differences in physical health states are obvious, preferences for health states are verifiable from surveys of patients and others, and in those instances where it is difficult to determine which of two health states is the more preferred, the two states can be given equal positions or ranks in the preference ordering. Nevertheless, since the issue is an empirical one and not susceptible to a definitive judgment, it will be maintained as an assumption throughout the book that, *both for individuals and the community as a whole, measured health benefits correctly order levels of health wellbeing.* Hence a GM health care agency that maximizes its community's total health benefits subject to its total cost constraint also produces a cost-constrained maximum of its community's aggregate health wellbeing. And by the same token, an MO agency that increases its community's total health benefits increases the community's overall health wellbeing.

Other issues indirectly associated with the measurement of QOL and health benefits bear on the utilitarian ethical foundations of CEA. Although it has its defenders, notably among economists, the utilitarian ethic has been a matter of dispute among philosophers since the time of Kant, and many of the criticisms of health benefits measurement and of CEA itself are special versions of centuries-old objections to utilitarian ethical theory. As has been said, patients can lose health benefits, even though the community's total quantity of health benefits is increased— when a new treatment is sanctioned for the health care agency's patients, a point first raised by Cantor [1994]. Other ethical criticisms of CEA are that

• Health benefits are not homogeneous. For instance, it can be argued that producing 20 QALYs for a seriously ill or disabled child is not equivalent to producing the same number of QALYs for 200 adults having minor back pains. Thus it is not necessarily true that a larger total quantity of health benefits implies a higher level of society's overall health wellbeing.

• The discipline fails to account for the dignity of individuals by not observing well established medical principles such as the rule of rescue (e.g., Eddy [1991], Hadorn [1991])—the principle by which one serious condition is given priority for treatment over perhaps a large number of more minor health problems.

   • Receiving health care is a basic human right that CEA ignores by failing to assure minimum quantities of health care to all persons having health problems.

   Although these criticisms bear on the ethical foundations of CEA, they can also be construed as claims that the instruments for measuring QOL and health benefits are improperly measured and aggregated. In CEA the community's health wellbeing is in effect defined as an unweighted sum of all patients' health benefits. Thus it is methodologically possible to deal with the measurement and aggregation criticism by attaching especially heavy weights to the health benefits received by those patients who are considered more deserving than others. Given their costs, the larger are the health benefits that treatments produce, the more likely are the treatments are to be given or made available to patients. Hence by attaching large enough weights to the QALYs received by serious or disabled children and by patients considered in need or urgent care, CEAs can be made to find absolutely cost-effective treatments for them. Similarly, instead of imposing constraints on the agency to force it to provide minimum amounts of care, the health benefits due to minimum-care treatment of the patient subpopulation or set of illnesses deemed deserving of minimum care could also be given sufficiently large weights so that CEAs will cause patients to be assigned to them.

   Although the strategy of weighting health benefits is a feasible one, deciding what the appropriate weights are or should be goes well beyond the purposes and capabilities of CEA. If the weighting of QALYs or other measures of health benefits is to become an integral feature of CEA, the work to make it so should be done by legislative or executive authorities and in conformity with societally accepted ethical standards. It is not a task for cost-effectiveness analysts. For that reason and because weighting systems for health benefits—whatever they are—does not affect the decision rules of CEA, they will not be considered in this book.

1.5 Health Care Costs in Cost-Effectiveness Analysis

Because the definition of the costs of treatments generally has no effect on the decision rules of CEA, it will be assumed that the definition has been made and is meaningful. It will be assumed, however, that every treatment cost is a constant and that the cost of every no-action treatment is zero. This latter assumption raises a much discussed issue in the literature on CEA. The issue concerns what is known as the proper "perspective" in which CEAs should be performed. A CEA can be conducted from two points of view, that of the health care agency *as payer* or that of the agency's community as a whole—its patients and non-patients alike. The latter is called the *societal perspective* and it differs from the payer's perspective in two ways.

First of all, if a CEA is performed from the perspective of the agency as payer, the costs of treatments are simply the actual money payments the agency makes to provide or insure those treatments for patients. They are usually called the *direct costs* of treatments. But when the CEA's perspective is societal, treatment costs include not only money payments to health care resource owners but also all other money and non-money costs the community incurs when patients are treated for illnesses. These other costs are chiefly those attached to the negative externalities or spillover effects of treatments for illnesses. In the literature agreement is mixed about which of these other costs should be recognized in CEAs, but the cost of unpaid caregiver labor services given by patients' families, patients friends, patients themselves, and perhaps by charities is often cited as a primary example. Hence from a societal perspective it can be argued that denying treatment for an illness causes the production of unpaid caregiver services that would otherwise be supplied by paid providers, and that these unpaid services are not costless to society.

The second way in which the societal perspective differs from the payer's perspective is that it values all costs at opportunity levels rather than at observed market levels or levels set arbitrarily by the health care agency. Since an opportunity cost is the maximum payment a productive resource would receive in any employment other than its given use, the claim is that the total opportunity cost of treatments is the largest value of other goods and services society gives up in order to provide health care for its patients.

By whatever means the costs of the negative externalities of paid health care—usually called *indirect costs*—are defined or specified, it is contended by many published authorities that the societal perspective is correct one for CEAs (e.g., Gold et al. [1996], Muennig and Khan [2002], Neumann [2009], Garrison et al. [2010]). The claim is that society as a whole is better off than it would otherwise be when it bears all of the costs of caring for its patients, not just those of money payments alone whatever they happen to be. The claim appears especially persuasive when the health care agency is publicly owned and its treatment costs are funded by taxes levied on the agency's overall community, since in that case some portion of the total cost of health care is already borne by the community at large.

Despite the facts that the welfare argument favoring a societal perspective seems overwhelmingly compelling and that there is no significant opposition to it in the literature on CEA, it will be assumed in this book that the model health care agency acts only with a payer's perspective. The reason for this is that the societal perspective either evokes the same kind of optimizing behavior as the payer's perspective or else it raises methodological problems that make CEA unworkable. To see that this is so, consider a GM health care agency that assumes a societal perspective. The agency will then attach indirect costs to the treatments it produces or insures, and it will value direct costs—money payments to providers—at opportunity levels. Next, though, the agency, its patient community, or some other authority must set constraints on total indirect costs and on the total opportunity costs of its treatments. If this is not done, the only constraint on the agency's choice of a global patient assignment is the constraint on the total money cost of its treatments. Hence the agency will seek to maximize its community's total health benefits subject only to this money payment constraint, and it would obtain the same optimal global assignment and total quantity of health benefits that it would if it ignored indirect and opportunity costs altogether. It would behave exactly as if it assumed a payer's perspective.

Suppose then that constraints on all costs, direct and indirect, are imposed on the agency and that they are valued at opportunity levels. How these constraints could be defined is not at all self-evident because there is no experience with selecting the maximum acceptable values of an agency's indirect costs or the opportunity values of its direct costs and there is no research or theoretical principle that might easily be used to choose them. But suppose these difficulties can be overcome, that constraints on its total opportunity and indirect costs are meaningfully chosen, and that the health care agency is required to function so as to meet them. Now if the agency is a global maximizer, it will attempt to maximize its community's total health benefits subject to the constraint on its total money treatments to its providers, and this constraint is either binding or it is not. If the constraint is binding, and whether the constraints on total opportunity and indirect costs are binding or not, the agency maximizes its community's total health benefits subject to the constraint on its total money treatment cost. That is, it ignores opportunity and indirect costs and behaves again exactly as if it takes a payer's perspective. On the other hand, if the money constraint is not binding because additional spending will force the agency to violate the constraints on indirect costs or opportunity costs, the agency violates

Weinstein's Axiom. It could but does not increase the community's total quantity of health benefits by spending on more or more health-benefit productive treatments. This conflict does not arise if money payments to providers are made equal to opportunity costs and are scaled to subsume the effects of indirect costs because in that case the money constraint on total money treatment cost is absorbed in the constraint on total opportunity cost. It seems unrealistic to think that an agency would and could behave in this manner, but if it does so it behaves once more exactly as if it assumes a payer's perspective. Money payments to providers equal the opportunity costs of formal health care and payments are preadjusted in some way so as cause the constraint(s) on total indirect costs to be satisfied.

To summarize the argument in a few words, the real or model health care agency faces a constraint on the total direct cost—its money payments to resource owners—of its treatments for its patients. This constraint is binding or it is not. If it is binding the agency necessarily acts with a payer's perspective. If the constraint is not binding, the agency cannot be a global maximizer and the foundation that justifies the decision rules of global CEA vanishes. The assumption of a societal perspective is therefore irrelevant to global CEA or else it nullifies the theoretical basis of the decision rules of global CEA. On these grounds it is assumed hereafter that the health care agency acts only from a payer's perspective. Finally then, and inasmuch as the agency pays nothing if it does not care for patients, it will also be assumed hereafter that the cost of the no-action treatment for every illness is zero.

1.6 The Information Requirements of Cost-Effectiveness Analysis

The usefulness of any decision-making procedure depends not just on its logic but also on the ease and cost of obtaining the data necessary for applying it, and this is especially true for CEA. The information requirements of CEA vary enormously depending on whether the scope of the analysis is global or single-treatment. For a global analysis—the assigning of all patients in the health care system to treatments for their illnesses—the analyst must know or have reliable estimates of:

- the cost of every treatment for every illness,
- the health benefits produced by every treatment for every illness,
- the total number of persons having each illness,
- the constraint on the agency's total (direct) treatment costs—the size of the agency's health care spending constraint.

The vastness of these information requirements shows why global CEAs have as yet rarely been performed.

The information requirements of single-treatment CEA conducted with either of the two health care agency models are many fewer. The methods of single-treatment CEA were developed by individuals and small groups of researchers who were neither employed by health care agencies nor members of agencies' organizations, and as a result these methods were designed to make use of the relatively little information that analysts could normally acquire or assemble. In the theoretical and empirical literature on single-treatment CEA it is customarily assumed that the analyst has three sets or items of information, and the same assumptions will be employed in this book. The information requirements are a knowledge or estimates of:

- the costs of all treatments for the particular or focal illness,
- the health benefits produced by all treatments for the particular or focal illness,
- the health care system's cutoff point.

It has already been said that for the purpose of deriving the single-treatment decision rules it will usually be assumed that treatment costs and health benefits are given data. The meaning and determination of the health care system's cutoff point will be discussed in subsequent chapters, but as it appears in the GM and MO models' decision rules it can be understood simply as the largest observed marginal treatment cost of producing health benefits in the agency's health care system. In practice the cutoff point or an estimate of it is ordinarily made by an outside authority and taken as a given datum by the analyst. But it can also be regarded as a parameter in single-treatment analyses, and when it is the analyst reports that a treatment is absolutely cost-effective if and only if the cutoff point is a ratio in a certain interval of values. It is then the agency's responsibility to ascertain whether its system's cutoff point is in that interval of values and to decide for itself whether the treatment is absolutely cost-effective for the focal illness.

References

Berger ML, Teutsch S.   Cost-effectiveness analysis: from science to application. Medical Care 2005; 43 (Suppl II), II49-II53.

Bowling A. Measuring Disease (2nd ed.) . Philadelphia: Open University Press, 2001.

Cantor SB. Cost-effectiveness analysis, extended dominance, and ethics. Medical Decision Making 1994;14: 259-26.

Coons SJ, Rao S, Keininger DL, Hays RD.   A comparative review of generic quality-of-life instruments.   Pharmacoeconomics 2000; 17: 13-35.

Coons SJ, Shaw JW. Generic adult health status measures, in Fayers P, Hays R (eds.) Assessing Quality of Life in Clinical Trials (2nd ed.) Oxford, UK: Oxford University Press, 2005.

Dijkers M.   Measuring quality of life: methodological issues.   American Journal of Physical Medicine and Rehabilitation 1999; 78: 286-300.

Drummond MF, O'Brien B, Stoddart GL, Torrance GW. Methods for the Economic Evaluation of Health Care Programmes (2nd ed). Oxford: Oxford University Press, 1997.

Drummond M, Sculpher M. Common methodological flaws in economic evaluations. Medical Care 2005; 43 (Supplement 7): II-5-II-13.

Eddy DM. Oregon's methods: did cost-effectiveness analysis fail? JAMA

1991; 266: 2135-2141.

Fayers P, Hays R (eds.) Assessing Quality of Life in Clinical Trials (2nd ed.) Oxford, UK: Oxford University Press, 2005.

Feeny D. Preference-based measures: utility and quality-adjusted life years, in Fayers P, Hays R (eds.) Assessing Quality of Life in Clinical Trials (2nd ed.) Oxford, UK: Oxford University Press, 2005.

Garber AM, Weinstein MC, Torrance GW, Kamlet MS. Theoretical foundations of cost-effectiveness analysis, in Gold MR, Siegel JE, Russell LB, Weinstein MC (eds.). Cost-Effectiveness in Health and Medicine. New York: Oxford University Press, 1996.

Garrison LP, Mansley EC, Abbott TA, Bresnahan BW, Hay JW. Smeeding J. Good research practices for measuring drug costs in cost-effectiveness analyses: a societal perspective: The ISPOR drug cost task force report—Part II. Value in Health 2010; 13: 8-113.

Gold MR, Russell, LB, Siegel JA, Weinstein MC (eds). Cost-Effectiveness in Health and Medicine. New York: Oxford University Press, 1996.

Hadorn DC. Setting health care priorities in Oregon: cost-effectiveness meets the rule of rescue. JAMA 1991; 265: 2218-2225.

Hays RD, Revicki D. Reliability and validity (including responsiveness), in Fayers P, Hays R (eds.) Assessing Quality of Life in Clinical Trials (2nd ed.) Oxford, UK: Oxford University Press, 2005.

Johannesson M, Weinstein MC. On the decision rules of cost-effectiveness analysis. Journal of Health Economics 1993; 12: 459-467.

Karlsson G, Johannesson M. The decision rules of cost-effectiveness analysis. Pharmacoeconomics 1996; 9: 113-120.

Klarman HE, Francis JO'S, Rosenthal GD. Cost-effectiveness analysis applied to the treatment of chronic renal disease. Medical Care 1968; VI: 48-54.

Laska EM, Meisner M, Siegel C, Stinnett AA. Ratio-based and net health benefit-based approaches to health care resource allocation: proofs of optimality and equivalence. Health Economics 1999; 8: 171-174.

Luce BR. What will it take to make cost-effectiveness analysis acceptable in the United States? Medical Care 2005; 43 (Suppl II), II44-II48.

Marshall JK, Cawdron R, Yamamura D, Ganguli S, Ladf R, O'Brien BJ.

Use and misuse of cost-effectiveness terminology in the gastroenterology literature: a systematic review. American Journal of Gastroenterology 2002; 97: 172-179.

Mishoe SC, Maclean JR. Assessment of health-related quality of life. Respiratory Care 2001; 46: 1235-57.

Muennig P, Khan K. Designing and Conducting Cost-Effectiveness Analyses in Medicine and Health Health Care. San Francisco: Jossey-Bass, 2002.

Neumann P. Costing and perspective in published cost-effectiveness analyses. Medical Care 2009; 47, Suppl 1: s28-s32.

Neumann PJ. Using Cost-Effectiveness Analysis to Improve Health Care. New York: Oxford University Press, 2005.

Neumann PJ, Greenberg D, Olchanski NV, Stone PW, Rosen AB. Growth and quality of the cost-utility literature, 1976-2001. Value in Health 2005; 8: 3-9.

Neumann PJ, Stone PW, Chapman RH, Sandberg EA, Bell CM. The quality of reporting in published cost-utility analyses, 1976-1997. Annals of Internal Medicine 2000; 132: 964-972.

O'Connor R. Measuring Quality of Life in Health. Edinburgh: Churchill Livingston/Elsevier, 2004.

Pauley MV. Valuing health care benefits in money terms, in Sloan FA (ed.). Valuing Health Care. New York: Cambridge University Press, 1995.

Phelps CE, Mushlin AI. On the (near) equivalence of cost-effectiveness and cost-benefit analysis. International Journal of Technology Assessment in Health Care 1991; 7: 12-21.

Russell LB. Cost-effectiveness analysis, in Chapman GB, Sonnenberg FA (eds.). Decision Making in Health Care. New York: Cambridge University Press, 2000.

Shepard DE, Thompson MS. First principles of cost-effectiveness analysis. Public Health Reports 1979; 94: 535-543.

Siegel JE. Cost-effectiveness analysis in US healthcare decision-making: Where is it going? Medical Care 2005; 43 (Suppl II), II1-II4.

Spiegel BMR, Targownik LE, Kanwal F, DeRosa V, Dulai GS, Gralnek IM, Chiou CF. The quality of published health economic analyses in digestive diseases: a systematic review and quantitative appraisal. Gastroenterology 2004; 127: 403-411.

Stinnett AA, Mullahy J. Net health benefits: a new framework for the analysis of uncertainty in cost-effectiveness analysis. Medical Decision Making 1990; 18 S68-S80.

Udvarhelyi IS, Colditz GA, Rai A, Epstein AM. Cost-effectiveness and cost-benefit analyses in the medical literature. Are the methods being used correctly? Annals of Internal Medicine 1992; 116: 238-244.

Weinstein MC, Fineberg HV. Clinical Decision Analysis. Philadelphia: WB Saunders, 1980.

Weinstein MC, Stason WB. Foundations of cost-effectiveness analysis for health and medical practices. New England Journal of Medicine 1977; 296: 716-721.

Weinstein MC, Zeckhauser R. Critical ratios and efficient allocation. Public Economics 1973; 2: 147-157.

2 Treatment Dominance

2.1 The Meaning of Treatment Dominance

Suppose n_A patients are initially assigned to treatment A for some illness. Then A is said to be *dominated* by one or more *dominating* treatments for the same illness if all n_A patients can be switched from A to the dominating treatment(s) and the new assignment costs no more than the initial assignment and produces at least as large a total quantity of health benefits. To state the concept of dominance more precisely, suppose there are J treatments, 1, 2,..., j,..., J, for an illness, and label the no-action treatment 1. Let N be the total number of patients having the illness, and let n_j be the number of patients assigned to or cared for by the j-th treatment. Let q_j denote the quantity of health benefits per patient produced by the j-th treatment, and let c_j denote the direct cost per patient of the j-th treatment. Assume that the cost and health benefit output of each no-action treatment are both zero and that the cost of every active treatment is positive. Formally then,

Definition: A treatment k for an illness is dominated if there exists a subset of treatments for the illness not containing treatment k, call it Q, and a set of positive weights α_j such that

(1)   all $\alpha_j > 0$, $\sum_{j \text{ in } Q} \alpha_j = 1$, $c_k \geq \sum_{j \text{ in } Q} \alpha_j c_j$, and $q_k \leq \sum_{j \text{ in } Q} \alpha_j q_j$,

and the treatments in Q for which (1) holds are said to dominate treatment k.

Definition: A treatment k for an illness is strictly dominated if at least one of the two inequalities

$$c_k \geq \sum_{j \text{ in } Q} \alpha_j c_j \text{ and } q_k \leq \sum_{j \text{ in } Q} \alpha_j q_j \text{ in (1)}$$

is strict.

There are exactly two kinds of strict and nonstrict ordinary treatment dominance. In the first of the two, treatment k is dominated by one or more single treatments. In the second, k is dominated by a combination of at least two other treatments one of which may be the no-action treatment. In the CEA literature the first type of dominance is usually called simply dominance, and the second type was named *extended dominance* by Cantor [1994] who first described it. Because it is awkward to describe a treatment as extendedly dominated or to say that it extendedly dominates another treatment, in this book the second type of dominance will be called *weak dominance* and the first type will be called *strong dominance*. A treatment may be both strongly and weakly dominated by other treatments, it may be strongly dominated by two or more single treatments, and it may be weakly dominated by two or more pairs of treatments. To economize on word usage, when a treatment is strongly dominated, weakly dominated, or both it will sometimes be said only that a treatment is dominated.

2.2 Finding and Removing Dominated Treatments from a Treatment Set: the Procedures

The first two propositions in this section give general tests for strong and weak dominance. The last three give a procedure for removing dominated treatments from a treatment set and a test by which the analyst can determine whether or not the set contains dominated treatments.

Proposition 1. (Strong dominance.) Assume that there are at least two active treatments for an illness. Then treatment k for the illness is strongly dominated by treatment m for the same illness if and only if

(2) $$c_k \geq c_m \text{ and } q_k \leq q_m.$$

Proof: Sufficiency follows by setting $\alpha_m = 1$ since in that case $c_k \geq$

c_m, $q_k \leq \alpha_m q_m$, and (2) therefore satisfies the defining condition (1) for treatment dominance. Necessity follows if there exist the inequalities $c_k \geq \alpha_m c_m$, $q_k \leq \alpha_m q_m$ with $\alpha_m = 1$ because these two inequalities are then identical to (2). The proof is now complete.

Remark 1. If treatment m dominates but does not strictly dominate treatment k, $c_k = c_m$ and $q_k = q_m$, and the two treatments are identical for the purposes of CEA even if they are not medically the same. *For that reason it will be assumed throughout the book that any two or more treatments that strongly but nonstrictly dominate one another are merged together into and regarded as a single treatment.* In this way nonstrict strong dominance can easily be incorporated into CEA, and if it happens that the composite treatment is found to be absolutely cost-effective, patients can be assigned at random or in any way the agency prefers to its constituent treatments. *Hereafter it should be understood that every strongly dominated treatment is strictly strongly dominated.*

Observe next that if all strictly strongly dominated treatments are removed from a treatment set, the remaining treatments can always be ordered and indexed so that treatment costs c_j and treatment health benefits q_j both increase strictly in the treatment index j. This is so because if there are a j and j-1 such that $c_j > c_{j-1}$ and $q_j \leq q_{j-1}$, j-1 strictly strongly dominates j, or if $c_j \leq c_{j-1}$ and $q_j > q_j$, j strictly strongly dominates j-1.

The following procedure can be used to identify and remove strongly dominated treatments from a treatment set.

1. Find all pairs of treatments k and m such that If $c_k = c_m$ and $q_k = q_m$. If there are two or more such treatments that nonstrictly strongly dominate one another, combine them and redefine the combination as a single treatment. Then all treatments remaining in the treatment set are either strictly strongly dominated or they are not.

2. Order the remaining members of the treatment set so that $c_j \geq$

c_{j-1} for j = 1, 2,..., J.

3. Begin the editing procedure with treatments 2 and 3. There are four possibilities:

- $c_3 > c_2$ and $q_3 \leq q_2$
- $c_3 = c_2$ and $q_3 > q_2$
- $c_3 = c_2$ and $q_3 < q_2$
- $c_3 > c_2$ and $q_3 > q_2$.

In the first pair of inequalities treatment 2 strictly strongly dominates treatment 3 by Proposition 1, and 3 should therefore be removed from the treatment set. In the second pair of inequalities treatment 3 strongly and strictly dominates treatment 2, and 2 should be removed from the treatment set. In the third pair of inequalities treatment 2 strongly and strictly dominates treatment 3, and 3 should again be removed from the treatment set. In the fourth pair of inequalities neither treatment strongly and strictly dominates the other and both treatments should be retained in the treatment set.

4. Go to treatment 4 and repeat step 3. If neither treatment 2 nor treatment 3 is deleted from the treatment set in step 3, compare treatments 3 and 4 as in Step 3. If $c_4 \geq c_3$ and $q_4 < q_3$, remove treatment 4 from the treatment set. If $c_4 \leq c_3$ and $q_4 > q_3$, remove treatment 3 from the treatment set. If $c_4 > c_3$ and $q_4 > q_3$, retain both treatments 3 and 4 in the treatment set. If either treatment 2 or treatment 3 is removed from the treatment set, rename the surviving treatment number 3 and compare it with the originally numbered treatment 4 as in Step 3. Retain both treatments in the treatment set if and only if $c_4 > c_2$ and $q_4 > q_2$.

5. Repeat step 3 sequentially for treatments 5, 6,..., J. When the procedure is completed, $c_j > c_{j-1}$ and $q_j > q_{j-1}$ for all j remaining in the treatment set. This condition, that the members the set can be ordered so that treatment costs and health benefits both strictly increase in the treatment index are used below to test for the existence of strongly dominated treatments in the set.

The next four propositions introduce a ratio that has a central role in the decision rules of CEA. It is called an *incremental cost-effectiveness (ICE) ratio*. Let A and B denote any two treatments for an illness neither of which strongly dominates the other. Denote their costs per patient and health benefits per patient by c_A, c_B and q_A, q_B, and because neither treatment strongly dominates the other it can be assumed that $c_A > c_B$ and $q_A > q_B$. *Then the incremental cost-effectiveness ratio defined or measured or calculated on treatments A and B is the ratio*

$$R_{AB} = \frac{c_A - c_B}{q_A - q_B}.$$

In words, the ICE ratio R_{AB} is the marginal or incremental cost of producing health benefits by switching patients from treatment B to treatment A, and the ratio is meaningful only if it is defined on treatments for the same illness, positive, and bounded from above. The *average cost-effectiveness (ACE) ratio* c_A/q_A is also a marginal or incremental cost of producing health benefits, but in this case health benefits are produced by assigning more patients to the same treatment A and not by switching patients from one treatment to another. The ACE ratio of the no-action treatment is not defined because $c_A = q_A = 0$.

Before continuing it is useful to have a lemma that characterizes relationships between ICE ratios:

Lemma 1. Assume that $c_p > c_k > c_m$ and $q_p > q_k > q_m$. Then if any one of the following inequalities holds the other two hold as well.

$$\text{(i)} \quad \frac{c_k - c_m}{q_k - q_m} \geq \frac{c_p - c_k}{q_p - q_k}$$

$$\text{(ii)} \quad \frac{c_k - c_m}{q_k - q_m} \geq \frac{c_p - c_m}{q_p - q_m}$$

$$\text{(iii)} \quad \frac{c_p - c_m}{q_p - q_m} \geq \frac{c_p - c_k}{q_p - q_k}.$$

Proof: It will be shown that (i) implies (ii), (ii) implies (iii), and (iii) implies (i). Suppose (i) holds. Then

$$(c_k - c_m)(q_p + q_m - q_m - q_k) \geq (c_p + c_m - c_m - c_k)(q_k - q_m)$$

whence

$$\text{(ii)} \quad \frac{c_k - c_m}{q_k - q_m} \geq \frac{c_p - c_m}{q_p - q_m}$$

and if (ii) is true,

$$c_k - c_p + c_p - c_m)(q_p - q_m) \geq (c_p - c_m)(q_k - q_p + q_p - q_m)$$

so that

$$\text{(iii)} \quad \frac{c_p - c_m}{q_p - q_m} \geq \frac{c_p - c_k}{q_p - q_k}.$$

Finally, suppose (iii) is true. Then

$$(c_p - c_k + c_k - c_m)(q_p - q_k) \geq (c_p - c_k)(q_p - q_k + q_k - q_m)$$

and this inequality gives

$$\text{(i)} \quad \frac{c_k - c_m}{q_k - q_m} \geq \frac{c_p - c_k}{q_p - q_k}.$$

The next proposition gives the conditions by which weakly dominated treatments can be identified in a treatment set.

Proposition 2. (Weak dominance.) Consider a set of treatments for a single illness. Then a treatment k belonging to this set is weakly dominated if and only if there exist (dominating) treatments m and p for the same illness such that $c_p > c_k > c_m$, $q_p > q_k > q_m$, and any of three inequalities holds:

$$\text{(i)} \quad \frac{c_k - c_m}{q_k - q_m} \geq \frac{c_p - c_k}{q_p - q_k}$$

$$\text{(ii)} \quad \frac{c_k - c_m}{q_k - q_m} \geq \frac{c_p - c_m}{q_p - q_m}$$

$$\text{(iii)} \quad \frac{c_p - c_m}{q_p - q_m} \geq \frac{c_p - c_k}{q_p - q_k}$$

Proof: The assertion will be proved only for the inequality (i) since it is then true for the inequalities (ii) and (iii) by Lemma 1. To establish necessity, suppose treatment k is dominated by treatments p and m. Then by the definition (1) of treatment dominance there exist an $\alpha_p > 0$ and an $\alpha_m = 1 - \alpha_p > 0$ such that

$$\alpha_p c_p + (1 - \alpha_p)c_m \leq c_k \text{ and } \alpha_p q_p + (1 - \alpha_p)q_m \geq q_k.$$

Since both inequalities cannot hold if $c_k < \min(c_p, c_m)$ or $q_k > \max(q_p, q_m)$, without loss of generality it can be assumed that $c_p > c_k > c_m$ and $q_p > q_k > q_m$. But in that case it follows that

$$\frac{c_k - c_m}{c_p - c_m} \geq \alpha_p \geq \frac{q_k - q_m}{q_p - q_m},$$

whence

$$\frac{c_k - c_m}{c_p - c_m} \geq \frac{q_k - q_m}{q_p - q_m},$$

and this inequality gives the inequality (i).

To prove sufficiency, suppose that $c_p > c_k > c_m$ and $q_p > q_k > q_m$ and the inequality (i) holds. Choose an ε so that

$$0 \leq \varepsilon \leq \frac{c_k - c_m}{q_k - q_m} - \frac{c_p - c_m}{q_p - q_m},$$

where the right-hand side of the inequality is non-negative by (i) of Lemma 1. Then set

$$\alpha_p = \frac{c_k - c_m}{c_p - c_m} - \varepsilon$$

and

$$\alpha_m = \frac{c_p - c_k}{c_p - c_m} + \varepsilon,$$

so that $\alpha_p > 0$, $\alpha_m > 0$, and $\alpha_p + \alpha_m = 1$. Now

$$c_k - \alpha_p c_p - \alpha_m c_m = c_k - c_p\left[\frac{c_k - c_m}{c_p - c_m}\right] - c_m\left[\frac{c_p - c_k}{c_p - c_m}\right] + (c_p - c_m)\varepsilon$$

$$= [c_k(c_p - c_m) - c_p(c_k - c_m) - c_m(c_p - c_k)]/(c_p - c_m) + (c_p - c_m)\varepsilon$$
$$= (c_p - c_m)\varepsilon \geq 0$$

because $p > m$. Hence $c_k \geq \alpha_m c_m + \alpha_p c_p$. Next,

$$q_k - \alpha_p q_p - \alpha_m q_m = q_k - q_p\left[\frac{c_k - c_m}{c_p - c_m}\right] - q_m\left[\frac{c_p - c_k}{c_p - c_m}\right] + (q_p - q_m)\varepsilon =$$

(3) $[q_k(c_p - c_m) - q_p(c_k - c_m) - q_m(c_p - c_k)]/(c_p - c_m) + (q_p - q_m)\varepsilon.$

36

Add and subtract $q_m(c_p - c_m)$ and $q_m(c_k - c_m)$ in the expression in square brackets. After rearranging terms the expression becomes

$$(c_p - c_m)(q_k - c_m) - (c_k - c_m)(q_p - q_m) - q_m(c_p - c_k) +$$
$$q_m(c_p - c_m) - q_m(c_k - c_m) =$$
$$(c_p - c_m)(q_k - q_m) - (c_k - c_m)(q_p - q_m) =$$
$$(q_k - q_m)(q_p - q_m)\left[\frac{c_p - c_m}{q_p - q_m} - \frac{c_k - c_m}{q_k - q_m}\right]$$

Thus (3) can be rewritten

$$q_k - \alpha_p q_p - \alpha_m q_m = \left\{\frac{(q_k - q_m)(q_p - q_m)}{c_p - c_m}\left[\frac{c_p - c_m}{q_p - q_m} - \frac{c_k - c_m}{q_k - q_m} + \varepsilon\right]\right\} \leq 0,$$

where nonpositivity follows because the first product inside the curly brackets is positive on account of $c_p > c_m$ and $q_p > q_k > q_m$, and the expression inside the square brackets is nonpositive by construction. As a result, $\alpha_m > 0$, $\alpha_p > 0$, $\alpha_m + \alpha_p = 1$, $c_k \geq \alpha_m c_m + \alpha_p c_p$, and $q_k \leq \alpha_m q_m - \alpha_p q_p$, and by the definition (1) treatment k is dominated by treatments m and p. This result completes the proof.

Treatment k is strictly dominated by treatments m and p if the inequalities in (i)-(iii) are strict. It has been remarked that if a treatment is dominated but not strictly dominated by one or more other treatments, the same quantity of health benefits can be obtained without changing total costs by assigning patients either to the dominated treatment or to the dominating treatments. The result is trivial if k is strongly but not strictly dominated, and if k is weakly but not strictly dominated it also follows immediately from (1) and Proposition 2. That is, if k is nonstrictly weakly dominated, it is dominated by two treatments p and m such that $c_p > c_k > c_m$ and $q_p > q_k > q_m$. Thus by (1),

$$\alpha_p > 0, \ \alpha_m > 0, \ \alpha_p + \alpha_m = 1, \ c_k n =$$
$$\alpha_p c_p n + \alpha_m c_m n, \text{ and } q_k n_n = \alpha_p q_p n + \alpha_m q_m n.$$

Because it is used in the chapters that follow, this result is stated as

Corollary 2. If treatments p and m nonstrictly weakly dominate treatment p, and n if patients are assigned to treatment k and to a pairing of p and m such that the total costs of the two assignments are the same, the total quantities of health benefits produced by the two assignments are also the same.

However, unlike the case with nonstrictly strongly dominated treatments, it is not possible to merge treatment k with treatments p and m that nonstrictly weakly dominate it and obtain a composite treatment having a well-defined cost and a well-defined product of health benefits. Suppose such a composite treatment is devised, let the numbers of patients assigned to k, p and m be n_k, n_p, and n_m, and let the cost and health benefit product of the assignment be c and q respectively. Then given n, n_k, n_p, and n_m must satisfy the equation system

$$n_k + n_p + n_m = n$$
$$c_k n_k + c_p n_p + c_m n_m = c$$
$$q_k n_k + q_p n_p + q_m n_m = q$$

The average cost and health benefit product of the assignment are $(c_k n_k + c_p n_p + c_m n_m)/n$ and $(q_k n_k + q_p n_p + q_m n_m)/n$, and for each n there are many different values of n_k, n_p, and n_m. Hence the average cost and health benefit product of the composite treatment vary with the distribution of the n patients among treatments n_k, n_p, and n_m, and there is no fixed unit cost or unit health benefit of the composite treatment.

When treatment k is weakly dominated, one of the two dominating treatments must be more expensive and more health-benefit productive than k, and the other must be less so. Accordingly, when the agency discards a weakly dominated active treatment as unsuitable for its patients, it reassigns patients to the two other treatments one of which produces fewer health benefits than k. This raises an ethical problem for the agency because it forces a decision as to which patients will receive the more health-benefit productive and which the less health-benefit productive of the two treatments. The problem becomes still more serious when the less health-benefit productive dominating treatment is the no-action treatment, for then the reassignment causes some of the patients who were formerly cared for by treatment k receive no care at all. This problem of fairness was first pointed out by Cantor [1994], and CEA has no mechanism for dealing with it. But as has been said, the aim of CEA is to cause the health care system to produce a larger than smaller total volume of health benefits for each given total health care cost. When some patients lose health benefits after a global reassignment the method by which the losers are redistributed to less health-benefit productive treatments is left to the health care agency.

The net benefits decision rules for single-treatment CEA discussed in Chapter 8 do not require that dominated treatments be identified and removed from the treatment set for the focal illness before they are applied. The rules have the convenient property that dominated treatments are simply ignored. However, the classical decision rules of single-treatment CEA do require that all dominated members of the treatment set for the focal illness before the absolute cost-effectiveness of a new treatment can be determined.

Several useful results follow when various types of dominated treatments are removed from a treatment set. Because they will be employed in subsequent chapters these results are summarized in

Proposition 3. Consider a treatment set for some focal illness.

(i) When all strongly dominated treatments are removed from the treatment set, the remaining members of the set can be ordered so that treatment costs c_j and health benefits q_j increase strictly in the treatment index j. (All strongly dominated treatments are strictly dominated.)

(ii) When all strictly dominated treatments are removed from the treatment set, the remaining members of the set can be ordered so that the c_j and q_j increase strictly in j and the ICE ratios

$$\frac{c_j - c_{j-1}}{q_j - q_{j-1}}$$

are nondecreasing in j.

(iii) When all strictly and nonstrictly dominated treatments are removed from the treatment set, the remaining members of the set can be ordered so that the c_j, q_j, and the ICE ratios

$$\frac{c_j - c_{j-1}}{q_j - q_{j-1}}$$

all increase strictly in j.

Proof: The claim (i) was established in the description of the procedure for removing the dominated members of a treatment set. The claim (ii) is true because if there are a j+1, j, and j-1 such that

$$\frac{c_{j+1} - c_j}{q_{j+1} - q_j} < \frac{c_j - c_{j-1}}{q_j - q_{j-1}},$$

Proposition 2(i) states that j is strictly weakly dominated by j+1 and j-1. The claim (iii) is true because if there are a j+1, j, and j-1 such that

$$\frac{c_{j+1} - c_j}{q_{j+1} - q_j} \leq \frac{c_j - c_{j-1}}{q_j - q_{j-1}},$$

j+1 and j-1 weakly but nonstrictly dominate j.

ACE ratios appear only infrequently in the decision rules of CEA, but is of some interest to see that when nondominated treatments are ranked so that the c_j, q_j, and

$$\frac{c_j - c_{j-1}}{q_j - q_{j-1}}$$

all strictly increase in j, the ACE ratios c_j/q_j also strictly increase in j.

Corollary 3.1 The ACE ratios c_j/q_j increase strictly (are nondecreasing) in all j if the members of a set of treatments are ordered so that the c_j and q_j strictly increase in j and, the ICE ratios

$$\frac{c_j - c_{j-1}}{q_j - q_{j-1}}$$

40

strictly increase (are nondecreasing) in j.

Proof: The proof is by induction on j. Since $c_1 = q_1 = 0$,

$$\frac{c_3 - c_2}{q_3 - q_2} > \frac{c_2 - c_1}{q_2 - q_1} = \frac{c_2}{q_2}$$

gives $c_3 q_2 > c_2 q_3$. Hence the claim is true for $j = 2$. Accordingly, assume the claim is true for an arbitrary j so that it must also be shown true for j+1—i.e., that $c_{j+1} q_j > c_j q_{j+1}$. But after simplifying,

$$\frac{c_{j+1} - c_j}{q_{j+1} - q_j} > \frac{c_j - c_{j-1}}{q_j - q_{j-1}}$$

gives

$$c_{j+1} q_j - c_j q_{j+1} > q_{j-1}(c_{j+1} - c_j) - c_{j-1}(q_{j+1} - q_j)$$

$$= q_{j-1}(q_{j+1} - q_j) \left[\frac{c_{j+1} - c_j}{q_{j+1} - q_j} - \frac{c_{j-1}}{q_{j-1}} \right]$$

$$> q_{j-1}(q_{j+1} - q_j) \left[\frac{c_j - c_{j-1}}{q_j - q_{j-1}} - \frac{c_{j-1}}{q_{j-1}} \right]$$

$$= \left[\frac{q_{j+1} - q_j}{q_j - q_{j-1}} \right] (c_j q_{j-1} - c_{j-1} q_j) > 0$$

by the induction hypothesis, and this result proves the claim for strictly increasing ICE ratios. Replacing the strict inequalities in the proof with weak inequalities proves the claim for nondecreasing ICE ratios.

An ordering relationship among ACE ratios will occasionally be referred to. It is this.

Corollary 3.2. In a set of nondominated treatments and $j \geq 2$,

$$\frac{c_j}{q_j} \leq \frac{c_j - c_{j-1}}{q_j - q_{j-1}}$$

with equality only if $j = 2$. That is, when they are defined, ACE ratios are never larger than ICE ratios.

Proof: If $j = 2$ the equality is obvious, and if $j > 2$ the strictly increasing monotonicity of ACE ratios

$$\frac{c_j}{q_j} > \frac{c_{j-1}}{q_{j-1}}$$

gives $c_j q_{j-1} + c_j q_j > c_{j-1} q_j + c_j q_j$. Thus $q_j(c_j - c_{j-1}) > c_j(q_j - q_{j-1})$, and this inequality proves the claim.

Propositions 1 and 2 show that strong and weak dominance exist, and It is clearly of importance to know whether there are other kinds of treatment dominance—and other kinds of treatments that are not absolutely cost-effective—as well. But, as has already been said, the answer is no. The next proposition, Proposition 4, states in effect that there are two and only two types of treatment dominance. The proof of the proposition requires another lemma, a proof of which is given in Appendix 2 at the end of the chapter. Although Lemma 2 is of no special importance in itself it is useful not only here but also in justifying the decision rules of CEA, and it will be referred to it many times in this and subsequent chapters.

Lemma 2. Suppose a treatment set contains J treatments. If $c_j > c_{j-1}$ and $q_j > q_{j-1}$ for all $j > 1$ and if

$$\frac{c_j - c_{j-1}}{q_j - q_{j-1}} > \frac{c_{j-1} - c_{j-2}}{q_{j-1} - q_{j-2}}$$

for all $j > 2$, then

(4) $$\frac{c_j - c_{j-1}}{q_j - q_{j-1}} > \dots > \frac{c_j - c_2}{q_j - q_2} > \frac{c_j - c_1}{q_j - q_1} \quad \text{for all } j > 2,$$

and

(5) $$\frac{c_J - c_j}{q_J - q_j} > \frac{c_{J-1} - c_j}{q_{J-1} - q_j} > \dots > \frac{c_{j+1} - c_j}{q_{j+1} - q_j} \quad \text{for all } j < J.$$

In addition, if $c_j > c_{j-1}$ and $q_j > q_{j-1}$ for all $j > 1$ and

$$\frac{c_j - c_{j-1}}{q_j - q_{j-1}} \geq \frac{c_{j-1} - c_{j-2}}{q_{j-1} - q_{j-2}}$$

for all j > 2, the strict inequalities in (4) and (5) are replaced with weak inequalities.

Proposition 4. The only types of treatment dominance are strong and weak dominance.

Proof: The proof shows that if a treatment set has no strongly or weakly dominated members, the assumption that it contains a treatment that is dominated in some third sense leads to a contradiction. So consider a treatment set that contains no strongly or weakly dominated members, and suppose treatment k is a member of the set that is dominated in some non-strong, non-weak manner.

Assume that the treatment or treatments dominating k comprise a subset Q of the given treatment set. Then by hypothesis Q contains no strongly or weakly dominated treatments, and by Proposition 3 it can be ordered so that treatment costs, treatment health benefits, and the ICE ratios defined on adjacent treatments in the ordering all increase strictly in the treatment index. Next, by Lemma 2 and the ordering of ICE ratios,

$$\frac{c_j - c_k}{q_j - q_k} > \frac{c_{k+1} - c_k}{q_{k+1} - q_k} > \frac{c_k - c_{k-1}}{q_k - q_{k-1}}$$

for all j in Q such that $c_j > c_k$ and $q_j > q_k$. The inequality relating the leftmost and rightmost of these ratios can be written

$$c_j(q_k - q_{k-1}) - q_j(c_k - c_{k-1}) + q_k(c_k - c_{k-1}) - c_k(q_k - q_{k-1}) > 0.$$

Multiply each of inequality by α_j and sum them. This gives

(6) $\quad (q_k - q_{k-1}) \sum_{j \text{ in } Q} \alpha_j c_j - (c_k - c_{k-1}) \sum_{j \text{ in } Q} \alpha_j q_j +$

$$\sum_{j \text{ in } Q} \alpha_j [q_k(c_k - c_{k-1}) - c_k(q_k - q_{k-1})] > 0.$$

In addition and also by Lemma 2,

$$\frac{c_k - c_{k-1}}{q_k - q_{k-1}} \geq \frac{c_k - c_j}{q_k - q_j}$$

for all j in Q such that $c_j < c_k$ and $q_j < q_k$., and this inequality can be written

43

$$c_j(q_k - q_{k-1}) - q_j(c_k - c_{k-1}) + q_k(c_k - c_{k-1}) - c_k(q_k - q_{k-1}) \geq 0.$$

Multiply each of these inequalities by α_j and sum them. The result is

$$(7) \qquad (q_k - q_{k-1}) \sum_{j \, in \, Q} \alpha_j c_j - (c_k - c_{k-1}) \sum_{j \, in \, Q} \alpha_j q_j +$$

$$\sum_{j \, in \, Q} \alpha_j [q_k(c_k - c_{k-1}) - c_k(q_k - q_{k-1})] \geq 0.$$

But from the definition (1) of dominance it must be true that

$$\sum_{j \, in \, Q} \alpha_j = 1, \; c_k \geq \sum_{j \, in \, Q} \alpha_j c_j, \text{ and } q_k \leq \sum_{j \, in \, Q} \alpha_j q_j.$$

Hence substituting these relations into (6) and (7) gives the single inequality

$$(8) \qquad (q_k - q_{k-1})c_k - (c_k - c_{k-1})q_k + [q_k(c_k - c_{k-1}) - c_k(q_k - q_{k-1})] > 0,$$

and the contradiction now proves the proposition.

Because the decision rules of CEA require that all dominated treatments be removed from the treatment set or sets in question before they are applied, it is useful to know when a treatment set contains no dominated treatments. Proposition 3 gives a necessary condition for the absence of dominated treatments—i.e., that the treatment set can be indexed and ordered so that the sequences of the c_j, q_j, and ICE ratios all strictly increase in the treatment index j—and as the next proposition shows, the same condition is also sufficient.

Proposition 5. A treatment set contains no dominated treatments if and only if it is possible to order and index the treatments so that the c_j, the q_j, and the ICE ratios

$$R_{ij} = \frac{c_j - c_{j-1}}{q_j - q_{j-1}}$$

all strictly increase in j.

Proof: Since Proposition 3 establishes necessity, it only needs to be proved that the treatment set contains no dominated members if the ordering premise is true. By Proposition 4 strongly and weakly dominated treatments are the only kinds of dominated treatments, and the treatment set therefore contains no dominated treatments if it contains no treatments of either of these types. So suppose the set of treatments can be ordered so that the c_j, q_j, and the ICE ratios

$$\frac{c_j - c_{j-1}}{q_j - q_{j-1}}$$

all strictly increase in j. If the treatment set contains a strongly dominated treatment, say treatment k, the definition of strong dominance and Proposition 4 imply that there must exist at least one other treatment m such that $c_k \geq c_m$ and $q_k \leq q_m$. But if $c_k \geq c_m$, treatment m must precede treatment k in the ordering, and in that event $q_m < q_{m+1} < ... < q_{k-1} < q_k$. Hence it cannot happen that $q_k \leq q_m$, and it follows that the treatment set cannot contain any strongly dominated treatments. So suppose instead that the treatment set contains at least one weakly dominated treatment k. Then by Proposition 2(i) there must exist an $m < k$ and a $p > k$ such that $c_m < c_k < c_p$, $c_m < c_k < c_p$, and

$$\frac{c_k - c_m}{q_k - q_m} \geq \frac{c_p - c_k}{q_p - q_k}.$$

However, the treatment ordering hypothesis and (4) and (5) of Lemma 2 give

$$\frac{c_k - c_m}{q_k - q_m} \leq \frac{c_k - c_{k-1}}{q_k - q_{k-1}} < \frac{c_{k+1} - c_k}{q_{k+1} - q_k} \leq \frac{c_p - c_k}{q_p - q_k}$$

for every $m < k$ and $p > k$, so that there cannot be any $m < k$ and $p > k$ for which

$$\frac{c_k - c_m}{q_k - q_m} \geq \frac{c_p - c_k}{q_p - q_k}.$$

This result proves that the treatment set cannot contain any weakly dominated treatments. Therefore, if the treatment ordering premise of the proposition holds, the treatment set contains no dominated treatments of any kind. This proves the proposition.

Proposition 5 provides a procedure for eliminating all dominated treatments from an initial treatment set for an illness. The procedure is this:

1. Order and index the treatments in the initial treatment set so that the c_j are nondecreasing in the treatment index j. This can be done for any treatment set. If there are tied values of the c_j, order the treatments within the group whose costs are tied in any manner, arbitrarily or at random.

2. In the ordered treatment set remove every treatment k such that $c_k \geq c_{k-1}$ and $q_k \leq q_{k-1}$ because all such treatments are strongly dominated. Ordinarily this step can be carried out by inspection and in one pass through the treatment set. When it is completed, the c_j and q_j of the remaining treatments must strictly increase in j.

3. Compute the ICE ratios on adjacent treatments in the (revised and) ordered treatment set. Beginning with treatment 1 and proceeding through the ordered treatment set, and if there is one, remove the treatment having the smallest index k such that

$$R_k = \frac{c_k - c_{k-1}}{q_k - q_{k-1}} \geq \frac{c_{k+1} - c_k}{q_{k+1} - q_k} = R_{k+1}$$

because k is weakly dominated by k-1 and k+1. Deleting k causes the deletion of the initial ICE ratios R_k and R_{k+1}, so before continuing, compute the new ICE ratio

$$\frac{c_{k+1} - c_{k-1}}{q_{k+1} - q_{k-1}}.$$

Then re-examine the treatment set and, if there is one, find the treatment having the next smallest index k' such that

$$\frac{c_{k'} - c_{k'-1}}{q_{k'} - q_{k'-1}} \geq \frac{c_{k'+1} - c_{k'}}{q_{k'+1} - q_{k'}}$$

because it is weakly dominated by k'-1 and k'+1. Remove k' from the treatment set, compute the new ICE ratio

$$\frac{c_{k'+1} - c_{k'-1}}{q_{k'+1} - q_{k'-1}},$$

and repeat the search and removal procedure until the ICE ratios in the ordered treatment set increase strictly in the treatment index. With that iteration, stop because all dominated treatments have been deleted from the treatment set.

This treatment editing procedure follows directly from Propositions 1, 2, 4, and 5. First of all, observe that it is impossible to delete a nondominated treatment from the treatment set because the tests in steps 2 and 3 cannot wrongly identify nondominated treatments. And although steps 2 and 3 are applied only to adjacent treatments in the ordered treatment set(s), it is also impossible to overlook and fail to delete a dominated treatment because the two steps together force a final ordering of treatments in which the c_j, q_j, and ICE ratios strictly increase in j, and by Proposition 5 the ordering implies that the treatment set contains no dominated treatments.

2.3 Removing Dominated Treatments from a Treatment Set: An Example

An example of the editing procedure for removing dominated treatments from a treatment set is shown in Tables 2.1-2.7. Suppose initially there are 11 active treatments for an illness. These are shown In Table 2.1 along with their costs per treatment c_j and health benefits per treatment q_j. The no-action treatment has been added to the treatment set and the treatments are ordered so that the c_j increase monotonically in j. Step 2 in the treatment editing procedure consists of identifying strongly dominated treatments and, if there are any, removing them from the treatment set. By inspection it is evident that treatments 5 and 6 are both strongly dominated—by treatment 4—and they are consequently removed from the treatment set. The first revised treatment set is shown in Table 2.2, and now there no other strongly dominated treatments in the treatment set because the costs per treatment c_j and health benefits per

Table 2.1
Identifying and Removing Dominated Treatments from a Treatment Set: The Initial Treatment Set

Treatment Number	Cost per Treatment (c_j)*	Health Benefits per Treatment (q_j)
1	0	0
2	4,000	2.5
3	8,000	4.5
4	8,500	5
5*	9,000	4
6*	10,000	5
7	12,000	6
8	16,000	6.5
9	18,000	7
10	22,000	8
11	23,000	8.5
12	25,000	9

*Strongly dominated treatment

Table 2.2
Identifying and Removing Dominated Treatments from a Treatment Set: The Treatment Set after the First Revision

Treatment Number	Cost per Treatment (c_j)	Health Benefits per Treatment (q_j)	ICE Ratio $\dfrac{c_j - c_{j-1}}{q_j - q_{j-1}}$
1	0	0	--
2	4,000	2.5	1,600
3**	8,000	4.5	2,000
4	8,500	5	1,000
7	12,000	6	--
8	16,000	6.5	--
9	18,000	7	--
10	22,000	8	--
11	23,000	8.5	--
12	25,000	9	--

**Weakly dominated treatment.

treatment q_j both strictly increase in j.

The final step in the treatment editing procedure is to search for and delete the treatments, if any, that are weakly dominated, and this is done by examining the sequence of ICE ratios. The rightmost column of Table 2.2 shows the ICE ratios calculated on adjacent treatments in the revised between treatments 3 and 4. Treatment 3 is therefore weakly dominated by treatments 2 and 4 and it is removed from the treatment set. Because a second revision of the treatment set is necessary after the removal of treatment 3, it serves no purpose to compute the ICE ratios on treatments 7-12, and they are omitted from Table 2.2. The second revision of the treatment set along with recomputed ICE ratios is shown in Table 2.3. Another reversal of the ordering of ICE ratios occurs between treatments 8 and 9, signifying that treatment 8 is strictly weakly

Table 2.3
Identifying and Removing Dominated Treatments from a Treatment
Set: The Treatment Set after the Second Revision

Treatment Number	Cost per Treatment (c_j)	Health Benefits per Treatment (q_j)	ICE Ratio $\dfrac{c_j - c_{j-1}}{q_j - q_{j-1}}$
1	0	0	--
2	4,000	2.5	1,600
4	8,500	5	1,800
7	12,000	6	3,500
8**	16,000	6.5	8,000
9	18,000	7	4,000
10	22,000	8	--
11	23,000	8.5	--
12	25,000	9	--

**Weakly dominated treatment.

dominated by treatments 7 and 9. After deleting treatment 8 the third revision of the treatment set is displayed in Table 2.4. In the table treatment 9 is found to be weakly dominated by treatments 7 and 10. Two more revisions of the treatment set are needed to identify and remove the weakly dominated treatments 10 and 11. These are shown in Tables 5 and 6, and the final edited treatment set is shown in Table 2.7. In Table

Table 2.4
Identifying and Removing Dominated Treatments from a Treatment Set: The Treatment Set after the Third Revision

Treatment Number	Cost per Treatment (c_j)	Health Benefits per Treatment (q_j)	ICE Ratio $\dfrac{c_j - c_{j-1}}{q_j - q_{j-1}}$
1	0	0	--
2	4,000	2.5	1,600
4	8,500	5	1,800
7	12,000	6	3,500
9**	18,000	7	6,000
10	22,000	8	4,000
11	23,000	8.5	--
12	25,000	9	--

**Weakly dominated treatment.

Table 2.5
Identifying and Removing Dominated Treatments from a Treatment Set: The Treatment Set after the Fourth Revision

Treatment Number	Cost per Treatment (c_j)	Health Benefits per Treatment (q_j)	ICE Ratio $\dfrac{c_j - c_{j-1}}{q_j - q_{j-1}}$
1	0	0	--
2	4,000	2.5	1,600
4	8,500	5	1,800
7	12,000	6	3,500
10**	22,000	8	4,000
11	23,000	8.5	2,000
12	25,000	9	--

**Weakly dominated treatment.

2.7 the editing procedure is complete because the c_j, q_j, and ICE ratios R_{ij} all strictly increase in j.

Table 2.6
Identifying and Removing Dominated Treatments from a Treatment Set: The Treatment Set after the Fifth Revision

Treatment Number	Cost per Treatment (c_j)	Health Benefits per Treatment (q_j)	ICE Ratio $\dfrac{c_j - c_{j-1}}{q_j - q_{j-1}}$
1	0	0	--
2	4,000	2.5	1,600
4	8,500	5	1,800
7	12,000	6	3,500
11**	23,000	8.5	7,333
12	25,000	9	4,000

**Weakly dominated treatment.

Table 2.7
Identifying and Removing Dominated Treatments from a Treatment Set:. The Treatment Set after the Final Revision

Treatment Number	Cost per Treatment (c_j)	Health Benefits per Treatment (q_j)	ICE Ratio $\dfrac{c_j - c_{j-1}}{q_j - q_{j-1}}$
1	0	0	--
2	4,000	2.5	1,600
4	8,500	5	1,800
7	12,000	6	3,500
12	25,000	9	4,333

2.4 A Geometric Interpretation of Treatment Dominance

The concept of treatment dominance is not a difficult one, and it can be grasped from diagrams as well as from algebra. For example, strong dominance is illustrated in Figure 2.1. In the figure the total health benefits Q produced by treating patients having an illness is measured on the horizontal axis. The total cost C of treating patients with the illness is measured on the vertical axis. Suppose that N patients have a particular illness, that there are many treatments for the illness and assume that two of them are initially labeled treatments 3 and 7. The point A represents the total health benefits and cost of treating $n \leq N$ patients having the illness with treatment 3, and the point B represents the total health benefits and cost of treating the same n patients with treatment 7. That is, the Q- and C-coordinates of A are q_3n and c_3n, and those of B are q_7n and c_7n. The cost and health benefit of the no-action treatment are $c_1 = q_1 = 0$, and these numbers are the coordinates of the origin. The slopes of the line segments OA and OB are the average cost-effectiveness (ACE) ratios c_3/q_3 and c_7/q_7, and the distances from the origin O to points on OA and OB are proportionally equivalent to the numbers of patients cared for

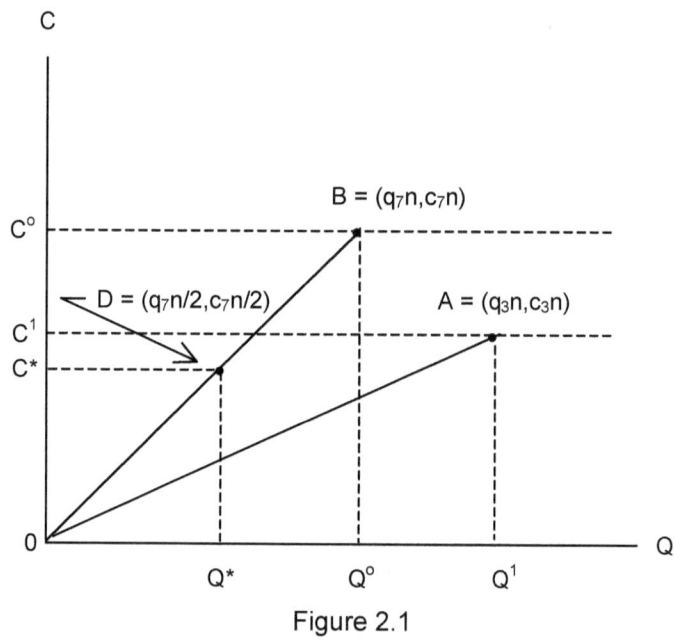

Figure 2.1

with the two treatments. For instance, the distance from the O to D on OB is one-half the length of OB, so that the Q- and C-coordinates of point D,

Q^* and C^*, are one-half the values of q_7n and c_7n respectively. Since q_7 and c_7 are constants, it follows that the number of patients given treatment 7 is $n_7 = n/2$ at point B.

Notice that $c_7 > c_3$ and $q_7 < q_3$, so that treatment 3 strongly and strictly dominates treatment 7 according to the condition of Proposition 1. But the result can easily be verified diagrammatically by comparing the coordinates of points A and B. Because $c_7 > c_3$, point A must lie below point B (i.e., $c_7n > c_3n$) and because $q_3 > q_7$ (so that $q_3n > q_7n$), point A must lie to the right of point B. Consequently, by "moving " from point B to point A—which is to say reassigning all patients having the illness from treatment 7 to treatment 3—the agency reduces its total cost of treating the illness from $C^0 = c_7n$ to $C^1 = c_3n$ and at the same time increases its total output of health benefits from $Q^0 = q_7n$ to $Q^1 = q_3n$. If the health care agency prefers to produce or have produced a larger than smaller total quantity of health benefits, it would therefore always assign patients to treatment 3 rather than treatment 7. Notice also that because n is arbitrary, the agency's action is the same regardless of the number of patients who are initially or might initially be assigned to treatment 7.

The second type of dominance, weak dominance, is depicted in Figure 2.2. Assume once more that there are many treatments for the illness three of which are originally labeled as treatments 2, 5, and 9. As in Figure 2.1 the coordinates of the point A are the total health benefits and total cost of caring for all $n \le N$ patients with treatment 2, and the coordinates of points B and D are specified similarly for treatments 5 and 9. Consider the line segments connecting A and B, B and D, and A and D. The slopes of these line segments are ICE ratios. For example, by inspection the slopes of the line segments AB and AD are

$$\frac{c_5 - c_2}{q_5 - q_2} \quad \text{and} \quad \frac{c_9 - c_2}{q_9 - q_2}.$$

Moreover, it is apparent that $c_9 > c_5 > c_2$, $q_9 > q_5 > q_2$, and

$$\frac{c_5 - c_2}{q_5 - q_2} > \frac{c_9 - c_2}{q_9 - q_2}.$$

Hence by Proposition 2(II) treatments 2 and 9 (strictly) weakly dominate treatment 5.

To see this relationship diagrammatically, first choose any point such as E on the line segment AB. The coordinates of E are $(q_2 n_2 + q_5(n-n_2)$, $(c_2 n_2 + c_5(n-n_2))$. They denote the assignment of n_2 patients to treatment 2 and $n-n_2$ patients to treatment 5 costing $c_2 n_2 + c_5(n-n_2) = C^1$ and producing $q_2 n_2 + q_5(n-n_2) = Q^1$ units of health benefits. But then there is a point G on the line segment AD having the coordinates $(q_2 n_2' + q_9(n-n_2'))$, $(c_2 n_2' + c_9(n-n_2'))$ and denoting an assignment of n_2' patients to treatment 2 and $n-n_2'$ patients to treatment 9. Moreover, the cost of the second assignment is

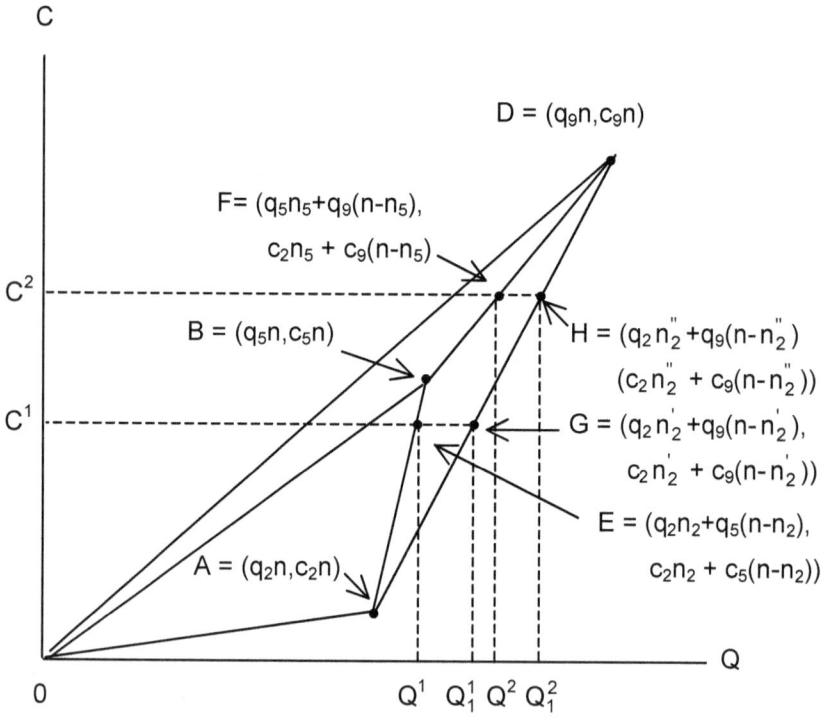

Figure 2.2

54

$c_2 n_2' + c_9(n - n_2') = C^1$ and the health benefit product of the assignment is $q_2 n_2' + q_9(n - n_2') = Q_1^1 > Q^1$ units. Hence the second assignment of n patients to treatments 2 and 9 costs the same as the assignment of n patients to treatments 2 and 5 but it produces a strictly larger quantity of health benefits.

An analogous result holds for equally costly assignments to treatments 5 and 9 and 2 and 9. Consider any point F on the line segment BD. It denotes the assignment of n_5 patients to treatment 5 and $n - n_5$ patients to treatment 9. The coordinates of F are $(q_5 n_5 + q_9(n - n_5), c_5 n_5 + c_9(n - n_5)$, the cost of the assignment is $c_5 n_5 + c_9(n - n_5) = C^2$, and the assignment produces $q_5 n_5 + q_9(n - n_5) = Q^2$ units of health benefits. But there exists another assignment of the n patients to treatments 2 and 9 denoted by the point H on the line segment AD and the coordinates $(q_2 n_2'' + q_9(n - n_2'')$, $c_2 n_2'' + c_9(n - n_2''))$. The assignment's cost is $c_2 n_2'' + c_9(n - n_2'') = C^2$ but its total health benefit product is $q_2 n_2'' + q_9(n - n_2'') = Q_1^2 > Q^2$. Thus in this case as well, it is possible to reassign patients from treatment 5 to a combination of treatments 2 and 9 so as to increase total health benefits without increasing total cost. Neither treatment 2 nor treatment 9 strongly dominates treatment 5 inasmuch as $c_9 > c_5 > c_2$ and $q_9 > q_5 > q_2$. Still, it is possible to switch patients from any assignment to treatment 5 to some combination of the two treatments 2 and 9 and thereby raise total health benefits without raising total cost. Hence the relationship between treatment 5 and treatments 2 and 9 depicted in Figure 2.2 is one of (strict) weak dominance of treatment 5.

Appendix 2   Proof of Lemma 2

Lemma 2. Suppose a treatment set contains J treatments. Then if $c_j > c_{j-1}$ and $q_j > q_{j-1}$ for all $j > 1$ and if

$$\frac{c_j - c_{j-1}}{q_j - q_{j-1}} > \frac{c_{j-1} - c_{j-2}}{q_{j-1} - q_{j-2}}$$

for all $j > 2$, then

(4) $$\frac{c_j - c_{j-1}}{q_j - q_{j-1}} > \ldots > \frac{c_j - c_2}{q_j - q_2} > \frac{c_j - c_1}{q_j - q_1} \quad \text{for all } j > 2$$

and

(5) $$\frac{c_J - c_j}{q_J - q_j} > \frac{c_{J-1} - c_j}{q_{J-1} - q_j} > \ldots > \frac{c_{j+1} - c_j}{q_{j+1} - q_j} \quad \text{for all } j < J.$$

In addition, if $c_j > c_{j-1}$ and $q_j > q_{j-1}$ for all $j > 1$ and

$$\frac{c_j - c_{j-1}}{q_j - q_{j-1}} \geq \frac{c_{j-1} - c_{j-2}}{q_{j-1} - q_{j-2}}$$

for all $j > 2$, the strict inequalities in (4) and (5) are replaced with weak inequalities.

Proof: Only (4) is proved because the proof of (5) follows closely similar lines. First of all, (4) is valid if

(9) $$\frac{c_j - c_{j-k}}{q_j - q_{j-k}} > \frac{c_j - c_{j-k-1}}{q_j - q_{j-k-1}} \quad \text{for all } k = 1,2,\ldots, j\text{-2}.$$

Furthermore, (9) holds if

(10) $$\frac{c_j - c_{j-k}}{q_j - q_{j-k}} > \frac{c_{j-k} - c_{j-k-1}}{q_{j-k} - q_{j-k-1}} \quad \text{for all } k = 1,2,\ldots, j\text{-2},$$

since from (9)

(11) $(c_j - c_{j-k})(q_j - q_{j-k-1}) - (c_j - c_{j-k-1})(q_j - q_{j-k}) =$
$\quad (c_j - c_{j-k})(q_j - q_{j-k}) + (c_j - c_{j-k})(q_{j-k} - q_{j-k-1}) -$
$\quad\quad (c_j - c_{j-k})(q_j - q_{j-k}) - (c_{j-k} - c_{j-k-1})(q_j - q_{j-k}) =$
$\quad (c_j - c_{j-k})(q_{j-k} - q_{j-k-1}) - (c_{j-kh} - c_{j-k-1})(q_j - q_{j-k}).$

Thus if (11) is positive, (9) holds and, in turn, this implies that (4) is true. To prove that (4) is true it is therefore sufficient to prove that the inequalities (10) are valid, and the proof of (10) is by induction on j. But (10) holds for $k = 1$ inasmuch as

$$\frac{c_j - c_{j-1}}{q_j - q_{j-1}} > \frac{c_{j-1} - c_{j-2}}{q_{j-1} - q_{j-2}}$$

by the strictly increasing monotonicity of the ordered ICE ratios, so assume that (3) is true for $k \geq 1$ and it must then be proved that (10) is also true for $k+1$.

That is, if

$$\frac{c_j - c_{j-k}}{q_j - q_{j-k}} - \frac{c_{j-k} - c_{j-k-1}}{q_{j-k} - q_{j-k-1}} > 0,$$

it must be demonstrated that

(12)
$$\frac{c_j - c_{j-k-1}}{q_j - q_{j-k-1}} - \frac{c_{j-k-1} - c_{j-k-2}}{q_{j-k-1} - q_{j-k-2}} > 0,$$

as well. But since the numerator and denominator of each of these two ratios is positive, the left-hand side of (12) has the same sign as

$$(c_j - c_{j-k-1})(q_{j-k-1} - q_{j-k-2}) - (c_{j-k-1} - c_{j-k-2})(q_j - q_{j-k-1}) =$$
$$(c_j - c_{j-k})(q_{j-k-1} - q_{j-k-2}) + (c_{j-k} - c_{j-k-1})(q_{j-k-1} - q_{j-k-2}) -$$
$$(c_{j-k-1} - c_{j-k-2})(q_j - q_{j-k}) - (c_{j-k-1} - c_{j-k-2})(q_{j-k} - q_{j-k-1}) =$$

(13)
$$(q_j - q_{j-k})(q_{j-k-1} - q_{j-k-2})\left[\frac{c_j - c_{j-k}}{q_j - q_{j-k}} - \frac{c_{j-k-1} - c_{j-k-2}}{q_{j-k-1} - q_{j-k-2}}\right] -$$
$$(q_{j-k} - q_{j-k-1})(q_{j-k-1} - q_{j-k-2})\left[\frac{c_{j-k} - c_{j-k-1}}{q_{j-k} - q_{j-k-1}} - \frac{c_{j-k-1} - c_{j-k-2}}{q_{j-k-1} - q_{j-k-2}}\right].$$

Consider the right-hand side of (13). The first difference in square brackets is positive by the induction hypothesis and the strictly increasing monotonicity of the ordered ICE ratios—i.e., because

$$\frac{c_j - c_{j-k}}{q_j - q_{j-k}} > \frac{c_{j-k} - c_{j-k-1}}{q_{j-k} - q_{j-k-1}} > \frac{c_{j-k-1} - c_{j-k-2}}{q_{j-k-1} - q_{j-k-2}}$$

and the second difference in square brackets is also positive by the strictly increasing monotonicity of the ordered ICE ratios. Each of the differences in the q_j is also positive by the strictly increasing monotonicity of the ordered q_j, and the difference (13) is therefore positive as well. This result verifies the induction hypothesis and completes the proof of (4).

With weak inequalities replacing strict inequalities, the same reasoning shows that

$$\frac{c_j - c_{j-1}}{q_j - q_{j-1}} \geq \ldots \geq \frac{c_j - c_2}{q_j - q_2} \geq \frac{c_j - c_1}{q_j - q_1} \quad \text{for all } j > 2$$

if $c_j > c_{j-1}$ and $q_j > q_{j-1}$ for all $j > 1$ and

$$\frac{c_j - c_{j-1}}{q_j - q_{j-1}} \geq \frac{c_{j-1} - c_{j-2}}{q_{j-1} - q_{j-2}} \quad \text{for all } j > 2.$$

This observation concludes the proof.

References

Cantor SB. Cost-effectiveness analysis, extended dominance, and ethics. Medical Decision Making 1994;14: 259-26.

3 Methods of Global Cost-Effectiveness Analysis

3.1 The Decision Problem in Global Cost-Effectiveness Analysis

In global CEA the health care agency's task is to assign every patient in its health care system to a treatment for the patient's illness. Hence the agency for whom global CEA is applicable chooses its global patient assignment in order to achieve some global objective. The myopic optimizer controls only a part, perhaps a very small part, of its health care system, and it is therefore not suited as a model for the conduct of global CEA. But the global maximizer's objective is to select a global assignment that maximizes its community's total health benefits subject to the agency's budget or treatment spending constraint. Hence the GM health care agency will be taken as the model agency for global CEA.

Again, the principal technological assumption in global and single-treatment CEA is that the costs and health benefits per treatment are both constants independent of the rate and scale of the production of treatments. The assumption also implies that the production of treatments is nonjoint—that is, the cost of each treatment is in no way affected by the rate and scale of production of any other treatment. It implies further that the outputs of health benefits are nonjoint, so that the health benefits produced by any treatment A are in no way affected by the volume of health benefits produced by another treatment B, even if B is intended for the same illness as A.

The constancy of unit treatment costs and health benefits allows the health care agency's total costs and total health benefits to be defined very simply. Respectively, let c_{ij} and q_{ij} be the cost and health benefit output of the j-th treatment for illness i, $j = 1,2,...,J_i$ and $i = 1,2,...,I$. Thus the cost of treating a patient with ij is c_{ij} and health benefits received by the patient is q_{ij}. Now let N_i be the number of patients having illness i and n_{ij} be the number of patients who are cared for by the j-th treatment for illness i. Then the total cost and health benefits attributable to all patients having illness i are

$$\sum_{j=1}^{J_i} c_{ij} n_{ij} \text{ and } \sum_{j=1}^{J_i} q_{ij} n_{ij}$$

respectively, and total cost and health benefits attributable to all patients having all illnesses are

$$\sum_{i=1}^{I} \sum_{j=1}^{J_i} c_{ij} n_{ij} \text{ and } \sum_{i=1}^{I} \sum_{j=1}^{J_i} q_{ij} n_{ij}$$

respectively.

Given the size of its spending budget C, the GM agency's objective is therefore to choose a set of treatments 11, 12,..., IJ_i for all $\sum_{i=1}^{I} N_i$ patients—a global assignment—that maximizes

$$\sum_{i=1}^{I} \sum_{j=1}^{J_i} q_{ij} n_{ij}$$

subject to the condition that

$$\sum_{i=1}^{I} \sum_{j=1}^{J_i} c_{ij} n_{ij} \leq C.$$

Mathematically then, the agency's decision problem is to maximize a linear function subject to linear constraints, and as a result it is natural to regard it as a linear programming problem. Although the global maximization problem was not then associated with CEA, the recognition that linear programming can be applied to find an optimal global patient assignment was first made more than 40 years ago by Torrance, Thomas, and Sackett [1972]. Hence the authors were also the first to propose, albeit implicitly, the GM model as the appropriate health care agency model for global CEA. Assuming the necessary treatment cost and health benefits data can be obtained, the fundamental problem of global CEA— finding a global patient assignment that maximizes the agency's community's total health benefits subject to a total spending constraint— can now be solved quickly with the use of inexpensive and readily available programming software.

A short discussion of the programming solution is given in the next section, but another method of solving the programming problem known as "prioritizing" has been developed in the past three decades and it is set out in Section 3.3. Two examples of the prioritizing procedure are then given in Section 3.4. Section 3.5 gives the principal implication of the prioritizing method for proving the decision rules of single-treatment CEA.

3.2 Solving the Decision Problem in Global Cost-Effectiveness Analysis by Linear Programming

Let total health benefits be written

$$\sum_{i=1}^{I} \sum_{j=1}^{J_i} q_{ij} n_{ij} = Q(n_{11}, n_{12}, \dots, n_{IJ_i}) = Q(n_{ij}).$$

Readers familiar with welfare economics will recognize $Q(n_{ij})$ as the simplest type of social welfare function—an additive or so-called Benthamite social welfare function (e.g., Johansson [1991]). A social welfare function is the aggregate utility of a given community or society expressed as a function of the quantities and conditions that produce or otherwise affect individuals' utilities. Hence the word "type" needs to be emphasized here because the health benefits q_{ij} are not to be interpreted as units of utility. That said, the decision problem faced by the GM health care agency is very much like that of the benevolent government in theoretical welfare economics. Given the constraints on its behavior such as the size of its resource base, the benevolent government seeks to organize its activities so as to maximize its community's total utility defined as a social welfare function. Similarly, the GM agency seeks to maximize its community's total health benefits $Q(n_{ij})$ subject *inter alia* to a budget constraint on its total costs.

Let C denote the agency's spending constraint budget, and let N_i be the total number of patients having illness i. Then the GM agency's decision problem—expressed as a linear programming problem—is this:

$$\begin{cases} \text{Choose the } n_{ij} \geq 0, \, j = 1, \, 2, \ldots, J_i, \, i = i, 2, \ldots, I \\[2mm] \text{To maximize } Q = \sum_{i=1}^{I} \sum_{j=1}^{J_i} q_{ij} n_{ij} \\[2mm] \text{Subject to the } I+1 \text{ constraints } \sum_{i=1}^{I} \sum_{j=1}^{J_i} q_{ij} n_{ij} \leq C, \, \sum_{j=1}^{J_i} n_{ij} = N_i, \, i = 1, 2, \ldots, I \end{cases}$$

(14)

Next, let the optimal total quantity of health benefits be expressed as a function of C: max $Q = Q[n_{ij}(C)] = Q(C)$. Let $c_{J_i} N_i$ be the largest total cost of treating patients with illness i, and let

$$\sum_{i=1}^{I} c_{J_i} N_i = C^T$$

be the largest total cost of treating all patients in the health care system. Then Q(C) is defined on the interval $[0, C^T]$ (inasmuch as it not rational to set a constraining total cost greater than C^T). The following statements are true.

(i) Q(C) is monotone strictly increasing on $[0, C^T]$.

(ii) Q(C) is concave and therefore continuous on $[0, C^T]$.

(iii) $\dfrac{\partial Q(C)}{\partial C}$ exists as a two- or one-sided partial derivative every-

where on $[0, C^T]$, is monotone nonincreasing in C, and is continuous except possibly at finitely many values of C.

Although general proofs of these properties of the optimal total health benefits function Q(C) require mathematics beyond the level of this book, most of them can easily be established from the prioritizing method, and that discussion will be deferred to Section 3.3.

In linear programming the formulation (14) is called a *primal program*. Every primal program has a symmetric *dual program* in which a decision variable is defined for each constraint in the primal program. In (14) there are I constraints requiring that the number of patients assigned to treatments for each illness i = 1, 2,..., I must equal the total number of patients having the illness, and one constraint requiring that total treatment cost cannot exceed C. Thus let $\pi_1, \pi_2, \ldots, \pi_I$ be dual decision variables associated with the first I constraints, and let π be the dual variable associated with the total treatment cost constraint. The dual programming problem of (14) is

(15)
$$
\begin{cases}
\text{Choose the } I+1 \text{ variables } \pi_i, \; i = i,2,...,I \text{ and } \pi \geq 0 \\[2mm]
\text{To minimize } \sum_{i=1}^{I} N_i \pi_i + C\pi = V \\[2mm]
\text{Subject to the } \sum_{i=1}^{I} J_i \text{ constraints } c_{ij}\pi + \pi_i \geq q_{ij}, \; j = 1,2,..., J_i, 1 = 1,2,...,I
\end{cases}
$$

According to duality theorem of linear programming, min V = max Q provided that a solution to either (14) or (15) exists (e.g., Dantzig [1963]).

The optimal values of the dual variables π_i and π are called the *shadow prices* of the constraint variables. That is, each of them is the marginal gain in optimal total health benefits max Q = Q(C) with respect to a marginal increase in the given constraint variable, and the shadow price of a constraint variable is zero if the constraint is nonbinding. The dimensions of π are not those of a conventional money price, but this is because Dorfman, Samuelson, and Solow [1958] who coined the term "shadow price" applied it to the each dual variable generated by a primal program in which the objective function is money-valued—either total profit or total cost—and in which the constraints are defined in physical units of productive inputs. In (14) by contrast, the objective function is defined in physical units and the constraint of principal interest, the total cost constraint, is expressed in monetary units. Let the shadow price of total cost C be expressed as the function $\pi(C)$. Then *$\pi(C)$ is the marginal gain in total health benefits with respect to a small increase in total cost C, and at the optimum it is understood as* $\dfrac{\partial Q(C)}{\partial C}$. Hence $\pi(C)$ is the reciprocal of a money price of health benefits—which is to say that it is expressed in units of health benefits per unit of money.

Because the health care agency is a global maximizer, it will be assumed that its total cost constraint is always binding at the optimum. Therefore, in the sense of Dorfman et al. the reciprocal of $\pi(C)$, $1/\pi(C)$, is the shadow price of health benefits relative to the agency's total spending constraint. It is, however, more readily thought of as a marginal cost. To see this, observe that $C(Q)$ is the inverse function of $Q(C)$, and because $C(Q)$ and $Q(C)$ are one-to-one and

$$\frac{\partial Q(C)}{\partial C}$$

exists, the partial derivative

$$\frac{\partial C(Q)}{\partial Q} = \left[\frac{\partial Q(C)}{\partial C}\right]^{-1}$$

also exists by the Inverse Function Theorem from classical mathematical analysis (e.g., Rudin [1976, p. 221]). Therefore,

$$\frac{1}{\pi(C)} = \frac{\partial C(Q)}{\partial Q}$$

is interpreted as the marginal cost of producing health benefits at the optimum. Moreover, because

$$\frac{\partial Q(C)}{\partial C}$$

is nonincreasing in C, the inverse function

$$\frac{1}{\pi(C)}$$

is nondecreasing monotonically in C, and as a consequence *the value of $1/\pi$ obtained from the dual program is the largest marginal cost of producing health benefits at the optimum.* Thus $1/\pi$ is both the GM agency's shadow price of health benefits *and also its cutoff point.* This last fact has no role in determining global patient assignments but it does have a central part in single-treatment CEA using the GM model. Because the connection between the global cutoff point and single-illness CEA is easier to describe in the context of the prioritization method, it is taken up in the next section.

That societal health care planning can be thought of as a routine problem in optimization theory has been remarked on by many authors since the publication of the model by Torrance et al., notably by Stinnet and Paltiel [1996] who present a number of programming variations of (14). Strictly speaking, in whatever way it is formulated, the maximization problem of global CEA should be solved by integer programming methods. But again for the sake of simplicity, in this chapter and in the rest of the book it will be assumed that the numbers of patients assigned to treatments can be varied continuously. The assumption entails a small loss of precision but, and this is especially true in the following chapters, having to deal with the n_{ij} as integer-valued variables adds complexity to the discussions without adding substance. The assumption is obviously most appropriate if the agency is large and the numbers of its patients are large.

3.3 Solving the Decision Problem in Global Cost-Effectiveness Analysis by the Prioritizing Method

While obtaining an optimal global assignment by linear programming has not always been described as a type of CEA, there exists a second method of solving (14) known as *the prioritizing procedure* that has explicitly been named a procedure of CEA. It has long been known that in global CEA the more health-benefit productive but more expensive treatments for illnesses become absolutely cost-effective and should be given to patients only as the agency's budget or the total cost of its resource base increases. And it has also long been known that the sequence in which these treatments become absolutely cost-effective as total costs increase is related to the ranking of ICE ratios (e.g., Weinstein and Fineberg, [1980]). In effect, then, this ranking of ICE ratios establishes a sequence or set of priorities by which treatments are offered to patients. The highest priority treatments—those that are offered to patients at small budgets or total costs—are those that increase the community's total health benefits with relatively small increases in total costs. Lower priority treatments—those offered to patients only at larger budgets or total costs—are those that increase the community's total health benefits but only at larger increases in total costs. Thus lower priority treatments replace high priority treatments in the agency's global patient assignment as the agency's budget or total resource cost increases.

Although the relation between treatment priorities and ICE ratios seems to have been intuited and partly understood by several other authors, the general prioritizing solution technique was first presented in its entirety by Karlsson and Johannesson [1996]. It was given, however, only by means of a numerical example without a proof of optimality, and the first proof of the optimality of the technique was published three years later by Laska et al. [1999]. That the prioritizing technique is, in fact, a method of solving the program (14) and consequently that the optimal global assignments obtained by linear programming and by the prioritizing method are identical follows from the fact that the prioritizing objective function and constraints are identical to those of (14). The prioritizing agency seeks to assign patients to treatments for all illnesses so as to maximize its community's total health benefits defined as

$$\sum_{i=1}^{I} \sum_{j=1}^{J_i} q_{ij} n_{ij}$$

subject to the condition that total treatment costs, defined as

$$\sum_{i=1}^{I} \sum_{j=1}^{J_i} c_{ij} n_{ij} \,,$$

cannot exceed the constraining value C and subject to the further conditions that all patients N_i having each illness i must be assigned to a treatment for the illness

$$\left(\sum_{j=1}^{J_i} n_{ij} = N_i \right).$$

These statements are the same as those of the programming problem (14), and they completely specify the decision problem addressed by the prioritizing technique.

As yet no software exists for obtaining global patient assignments by the prioritization method. Thus In view of the ease with which (14) can be solved and a global assignment obtained by inexpensive and readily available programming software, it is appropriate to ask why a agency or analyst should choose the prioritization method rather than linear programming for solving its optimization problem. One explanation is that the prioritizing procedure generates the set of optimal, absolutely cost-effective treatments for every total cost C, and this treatment set can be of interest to health care authorities or others having concerns about the priorities attached to these treatments. Obviously, linear programming can generate the same sets as well, but only by solving the optimization problem (14) iteratively for different values of C.

All the same, here the main reason for presenting the prioritizing technique is theoretical. The standard decision rules of single-treatment CEA can be deduced from the prioritization technique but not, or at least not easily, from the mechanisms of linear programming. Introducing a new activity such as assigning a number of patients to a treatment for a new illness is a common kind of programming problem, but it is solved by means of manipulations of the matrix of optimal coefficients obtained from the solution of the initial program (e.g., Danzig and Thapa [1997, pp. 184-85]), the matrix of coefficients that, when multiplied by the N_1, N_2,..., N_I expressed as a vector, yields the agency's initial optimal global patient assignment. These manipulations present no difficulties for a GM agency that has programmed the initial optimal global patient assignment, but an analyst having to decide whether or not a new treatment should be offered to patients is unlikely to possess even a small portion of the information—all treatment costs, all treatment health benefits, the numbers of patients having all illnesses, and the constraining total cost C—necessary to make the computations. The special strength of single-treatment CEA is that it does not require this huge body of information, and until advances in the theory of linear programming make it possible to obtain the single-treatment decision rules from the conventional methods for solving (14), these rules are most easily derived from the prioritizing technique.

The simplest version of the prioritizing technique and the only one ever intended for real-world health care planning was designed by the Oregon State Health Commission (OHSC) in 1989-90 and meant as a guide for allocating funds in the state's Medicaid program. The OSHC constructed a set of roughly 709 "condition-treatment pairs"—what are called illnesses here—many of which were congeries of conditions for related but nonidentical medical problems. It recruited physicians to define the possible health outcomes of caring for these condition-treatment pairs or illnesses and to specify the probabilities of occurrence of the outcomes. The costs of the outcomes were taken from Medicaid claims data or estimated by the physicians, and the expected cost of each treatment was defined as the sum of outcome costs weighted by the probabilities of their occurrence. Physicians also estimated the durations of treatment effects. To estimate the health benefits of the treatments, the OHSC assigned a health state to each medical outcome using the Quality of Well-Being Scale constructed by Kaplan and Anderson [1988, 1990]. The Commission then conducted a telephone survey of 1,001 non-physician residents of Oregon and asked the respondents to rate the health states from 0 (for death) to 1 (for perfect health). The expected number of health-state adjusted years of life for each treatment was next estimated as the duration of the treatment effect times the sum of the products of the rated health states and the probabilities of their occurrences. Finally, the net expected number of health-state adjusted years of life for each treatment was defined as this last figure minus the (similarly evaluated) number of health-state adjusted years of life if no treatment had been performed.

The OHSC recognized only two alternatives for each illness/condition-treatment, treat or do not treat. Hence in the terminology used here the OHSC defined only two treatments for each illness, one active treatment and the no-action treatment. The cost per treatment (or patient) for each illness $i = 1, 2,..., I (= 709)$ was the money cost to the Medicaid program c_i, and health benefits per treatment q_i was the net health benefit gained from treatment versus no treatment. The costs and health benefits of all no-action treatments were both set at zero. It is not clear how the OHSC derived the number of patients having or expected to have each illness, although the figures would not be difficult to estimate from historical Medicaid claims data. In any case, the Commission calculated the total cost and total health benefits of each treatment i as $c_i N_i$ and $q_i N_i$ respectively.

Given these assumptions the planning problem formulated by the Commission was how to assign Medicaid patients to its condition-treatment pairs so as to maximize the Medicaid population's total health benefits subject to the Medicaid budget constraint. Let C denote that constraint, and let n_i denote the number of patients having illness i who are to be treated. In the OHSC's formulation of its decision problem the health benefits ascribed to each patient having illness i was defined as $q_i = q_i^+ + q_i^-$ where q_i^+ stands for the health benefit if the patient is treated and q_i^- stands for the benefits if the patient is not treated. The formulation conflicts the argument given in Chapter 1 that patients' losses of health benefits should not be debited against the agency. (For that matter it is not immediately clear why it should be that $q_i^+ \neq q_i^-$, and if $q_i^+ = q_i^-$ the decision problem becomes meaningless.) However, the OHSC did assume that the costs of not treating patients were zero. In any case, the cost of actively treating n_i patients having illness i is $c_i n_i$, and if I* is the number of illnesses that are cared for (all patients having illnesses I*+1, I*+2,...,I receive no-action treatments), the total cost of treating all patients is

$$\sum_{1=1}^{I^*} c_i n_i = \sum_{1=1}^{I} c_i n_i ,$$

and total health benefits is

$$\sum_{i=1}^{I^*} q_i n_i = \sum_{i=1}^{I} (q_i^+ - q_i^-) n_i .$$

The optimizing problem facing a GM agency like the OHSC can then be stated in this way:

(16)
$$\begin{cases} \text{Choose the } n_1, n_2, ..., n_I \geq 0 \\ \text{To maximize } Q = \sum_{i=1}^{I} q_i n_i \\ \text{Subject to the } I+1 \text{ constraints } \sum_{i=1}^{I} c_i n_i \leq C \text{ and } n_i \leq N_i, \\ \qquad\qquad\qquad\qquad\qquad\qquad\qquad\qquad i = 1, 2, ..., I \end{cases}$$

In linear programming this kind of optimizing problem is known as a bounded variable problem, but it is easily solved without the use of a programming algorithm. To see that, calculate the average cost-effectiveness (ACE = ICE) ratio for each active treatment and order and index the ratios from smallest to largest. If there are one or more groups of treatments for which the ACE ratios equal, order and index the treatments within each group arbitrarily or at random. Because there is exactly one active treatment per illness the ordering of ACE ratios then imposes an ordering on illnesses as well as treatments. Let 1 denote the smallest ACE ratio and the first illness (or treatment) in the ordered set of all illnesses (or treatments), 2 denote the next smallest ACE ratio and the second illness (or treatment) in the ordered set of illnesses (or treatments), and so on for i = 3,4,...I. Now let I*, 0 < I* ≤ I, be the index of the largest ACE ratio such that

$$\sum_{i=1}^{I^*} c_i N_i \leq C .$$

Then the optimal global patient assignment is given by

Proposition 7. For (16) it is optimal to set $n_i = N_i$ for i = 1,2,..., I*-1,

$$n_{I^*} = (C - \sum_{i=1}^{I^*-1} c_i N_i)/c_{I^*}, \text{ and } n_i = 0 \text{ for } i = I^*+1, I^*+2,..., I.$$

Proof: The claimed optimal global assignment exhausts the

70

agency's budget (or the total cost of its treatment resources). Thus the only possible way to obtain a larger total quantity of health benefits than the quantity produced by the claimed optimal global assignment is to revise the global assignment so that at least some patients who are not cared for are reassigned to active treatments and some patients who are cared for are reassigned to no-action treatments. Therefore suppose $k > I^* \geq i$ and Δn_k patients cared for by a treatment having the k-th ACE-ratio rank are switched with Δn_i patients cared for by a treatment having the i-th ACE-ratio rank so as to preserve the constancy of total costs. Then $\Delta n_i c_i = \Delta n_k c_k$. But since

$$\frac{c_k}{q_k} \geq \frac{c_i}{q_i},$$

it follows that

$$\frac{\Delta n_k c_k}{\Delta n_k q_k} \geq \frac{\Delta n_i c_i}{\Delta n_i q_i} = \frac{\Delta n_k c_k}{\Delta n_i q_i} \text{ and } \Delta n_i q_i \geq \Delta n_k q_k.$$

Accordingly, any shift of patients between a treatment ranked higher than I^* and one ranked equal to or lower than I^* that does not change total treatment costs either reduces or does not change total health benefits. The claimed optimal patient assignment must therefore be optimal.

Although it did not publish a rigorous statement or proof of its assignment procedure, the OHSC apparently intended to use the method of Proposition 7 to make treatments available to Medicaid patients. All patients having illnesses indexed 1,2,..., I^*-1 and

$$n_{i^*} = (C - \sum_{1=1}^{I^*-1} c_i N_i)/c_{i^*} \leq N_i$$

patients having the illness indexed I^* would be cared for, but no other patients would be treated. Hence the illnesses indexed 1,2,...,I^* were given the agency's highest treatment priorities and illnesses indexed I^*+1, $I^*+2,...,I$ were given the lowest.

The OHSC's assignment procedure was widely characterized as CEA and as a scheme for prioritizing health care, and it was immediately and vigorously criticized on both technical and ethical grounds. In some instances it became evident that the OHSC's staff had combined two or more noncomparable medical problems in order to create a single condition-treatment pair, and in a number of other instances treatment costs and health benefits were not accurately or even plausibly estimated. But the most ardent criticisms were of the principles of CEA some of which are described in Chapter 1. It was argued that the OHSC's health plan amounted to rationing health care for the poor (despite the obvious fact that rationing of some kind—even by private market pricing mechanisms—is inevitable whenever patients cannot freely obtain all of the health care they demand), that the loss of health benefits due to one loss of life cannot be offset by the gains of health benefits by patients treated successfully for non-life-threatening conditions, and that the proper ranking of illnesses should be made by their social value instead of by their health benefits per dollar of cost. By the early 1990s these kinds of criticisms caused the OHSC to abandon the CEA methodology and replace it with a subjectively determined, three-tier classification of the original 709 condition-treatment pairs that were divided into 17 broad categories and ranked from "essential" (highest priority) to "basic" (lowest priority). And still later in 1993 Medicaid patients having only the highest ranked 587 condition-treatment pairs were made eligible for care. For various comments on the OHSC's experiment in global CEA see Eddy [1991], Hadorn [1991], Weiner [1992], Fox and Leichter [1993], Kitzhaber [1993], Kaplan [1994], and Blumstein [1997].

The prioritizing procedure for solving the global assignment problem (16) in which there is only one active treatment per illness is a special case of the Karlsson–Johannesson prioritizing procedure for solving the general global assignment problem in which there are two or more active treatments for at least some illnesses. Although Laska et al. [1999] have given a proof of the optimality of the procedure, their formulation of the optimal global assignment is not useful for deriving the decision rules of single-treatment CEA. For that reason the optimal global patient assignment obtained by the prioritizing procedure is stated below in a form from which the GM decision rules of single-treatment CEA are developed in Chapter 4.

To find the assignment and prove its optimality, several preparatory steps must be undertaken. These are:

1. Remove all dominated treatments from the every treatment set for every illness.

2. Order and index the remaining treatments for each illness i so that the c_{ij} (or q_{ij}) increase strictly in j.

3. Compute the ICE ratios

$$R_{ij} = \frac{c_{ij} - c_{ij-1}}{q_{ij} - q_{ij-1}}$$

on adjacent treatments in each of the ordered treatment sets. By Proposition 5 the treatments for each illness are then ordered so that the c_{ij}, q_{ij}, and R_{ij} all strictly increase in the index j.

4. Rank the ICE ratios for all treatments for all illnesses from smallest to largest. If there are one or more groups of equal ICE ratios, order the ratios within each such group arbitrarily or at random. Assign the rank number 1 to the smallest of all of the ICE ratios, 2 to the next smallest ICE ratio, and so on. The rank numbers attached to ICE ratios within the groups where the ratios are equal will vary with the ordering. The total number of ICE ratios equals the total number of active treatments.

5. Let the ranked ICE ratios be indexed by $t = 1,2,\ldots, T$, and let ρ_{ij}^t be the rank number of the t-th ICE ratio. The subscript ij means that the t-th ratio in the ranked set is R_{ij}. Notice that $R_{ij} > R_{hk}$ implies $\rho_{ij}^t > \rho_{hk}^s$ and t > s. But $\rho_{ij}^t > \rho_{hk}^s$ implies only that $R_{ij} \geq R_{hk}$ since if $R_{ij} = R_{hk}$, R_{ij} can be given a higher or lower rank number than R_{hk}. The fact that any two equal ICE ratios can be ordered so that either of them has a higher rank number than the other enters into the derivations and proofs of some of the single-treatment decision rules of Chapter 4.

Definition. Consider the set of T+1 total treatment costs C^t, t = 0, 1,...,T. These will be called *budget points*. The definition of C^t is this:

(17) $C^t = \begin{cases} 0 \text{ if } t = 0 \\ C^{t-1} + (c_{ij} - c_{ij-1})N_i \text{ if } t \geq 1 \text{ and } \rho^t = R_{ij}, \ 2 \leq j \leq J_i, \ i = 1 \leq i \leq I \end{cases}$

By this definition each budget point t > 0 is uniquely associated with an ICE ratio R_{ij} and with the rank number ρ_{ij}^t of that ICE ratio. Therefore it is also uniquely associated with the two treatments ij and ij-1 that define R_{ij}.

Definition. The set of all budget points generates an ordered set of T+1 intervals of total costs that will be called *budget intervals*. Define the 0-th budget interval as the single total cost [0] and the budget intervals for $t \geq 1$ as $(0, C^1], (C^1, C^2], ..., (C^{t-1}, C^t], ..., (C^{T-1}, C^T]$ where

$$C^T = \sum_{i=1}^{I} c_{iJ_i} N_i$$

is the total cost of treating all illnesses. The set of all total costs is the interval $[0, C^T]$, and it is the set union of all budget intervals. Because budget intervals are contiguous and disjoint, every total cost C is a point in exactly one budget interval. Each budget interval $(C^{t-1}, C^t]$ is uniquely associated with the budget point C^t, and by that token it is uniquely associated with the rank number ρ_{ij}^t of an ICE ratio R_{ij} and with the treatments ij and ij-1 that define R_{ij}.

Notice that the ordering of budget intervals from left to right (by the values of t) on $[0, C^T]$ is one-to-one with the ordering of ICE ratios—with the rank numbers ρ_{hk}. That is, if R_{hk} is associated with the budget interval $(C^{s-1}, C^s]$, and R_{ij} is associated with the budget interval $(C^{t-1}, C^t]$, $\rho_{hk}^s <$ ρ_{ij}^t, if and only if $(C^{s-1}, C^s]$ is positioned to the left of $(C^{t-1}, C^t]$—i.e., $C^s \leq$ C^{t-1}—in the ordered set of all budget intervals. This fact will be used in Chapter 4. Except when it is essential to show the exact positions of ICE ratios in the ordered set of all ICE ratios the superscripts on the ρ_{ij} will hereafter be omitted. The budget interval [0] is uniquely associated with all I no-action treatments, and if the budget interval $(C^{s-1}, C^s]$ is associated with treatment hk and hk-1, the length of $(C^{s-1}, C^s]$ is $(c_{hk} - c_{hk-1})N_h$. The lengths of budget intervals have an important part in the derivation of the single-treatment CEA decision rules of Chapter 4.

The final step necessary to perform the prioritization procedure is this.

6. Compute all budget points $C^1, C^2, ..., C^T$ and construct all of the budget intervals $(C^{t-1}, C^t]$.

Assuming that steps 1-6 on the initial global treatment set have been carried out, the GM health care agency's optimal global patient assignment is stated in

Proposition 8. The Optimal Treatment Prioritizing Policy. Let $n_{hk}(C)$ be the optimal (cost-constrained, health-benefit-maximizing) number of patients assigned to the k-th treatment for the h-th illness when the total cost of all treatments is C and

$$\sum_{k=1}^{K} n_{hk}(C) = N_h.$$

If $t = 0$ and $C = 0$, $n_{h1}(C) = N_h$ and $n_{hk}(C) = 0$ for all $k > 1$. If $C^t > 0$, C is a total cost in the budget interval $(C^{t-1}, C^t]$, and the interval is associated with R_{ij} and the rank number ρ_{ij}. Then for this one illness i,

$$(18) \qquad \begin{cases} n_{ij}(C) = (C - C^{t-1})/(c_{ij} - c_{ij-1}) \\ n_{ij-1}(C) = N_i - n_{ij}(C) \\ n_{ik}(C) = 0 \text{ for all } k \neq j, ij-1 \end{cases}.$$

Now consider every other illness $h \neq i$. Define treatment hk(h) so that

$$(19) \qquad hk(h) = \begin{cases} h1 \text{ if } R_{h2} > R_{ij} \\ \text{such that } \rho_{hk(h)} = \max_m \{\rho_{hm} < \rho_{ij}\} \text{ otherwise} \end{cases}.$$

Then for each such $h \neq i$,

$$(20) \qquad n_{hk}(C) = \begin{cases} N_h \text{ if } k = k(h) \\ 0 \text{ if } k \neq k(h) \end{cases}.$$

The formulation of the optimal global decision rules may seem complicated but the rules are easy to apply. The first step is to identify the budget interval from among the ordered set of all budget intervals that contains C. That interval is uniquely associated with an ICE ratio R_{ij} and with the treatments ij and ij-1. The optimal values of n_{ij} and n_{ij-1} are then determined from (18). Next and for each illness $h \neq i$, find the highest-ranked ICE ratio R_{hk} defined on the ordered treatments for h that is no larger than R_{ij}. If there is no such ratio, it is optimal to assign all patients having h to the no–action treatment h1. But if $R_{h2} < R_{ij}$, it is optimal to assign all patients having h to hk = hk(h). In practice it is probably most helpful to determine the optimal assignment by first constructing a table of the ordered sets of ICE ratios and budget intervals. This has been done for the numerical examples of prioritization given in Section 3.4 and in Chapter 6.

Proof of Proposition 8: What will be proved is that given C no other global assignment produces a larger total quantity of health benefits than the global assignment (18)-(20). The optimality of $n_{h1}(C) = N_i$ and all other $n_{hk}(C) = 0$ is trivial when C = 0, so assume that C > 0. Then as just said C is in some budget interval $(C^{t-1}, C^t]$ that is associated with the ICE ratio R_{ij}. By (18)-(20) the optimal total health benefits produced by treating illness i is

(21) $\quad Q(C) = q_{ij}n_{ij} + q_{ij-1}n_{ij-1} + \sum_{h \neq i} q_{hk(h)}N_h = (q_{ij} - q_{ij-1})n_{ij}(C) + \sum_h q_{hk(h)}N_h$,

where ik(i) = ij in the last sum on the right. Similarly, the total cost of the claimed optimal global assignment is

$$C = (c_{ij} - c_{ij-1})n_{ij}(C) + \sum_h c_{hk(h)}N_h .$$

Now let (n'_{hk}) be any other global assignment costing no more than C. The total health benefits produced by the second assignment is

$$Q = \sum_h \sum_k q_{hk}n'_{hk} ,$$

and the total cost of the assignment is

$$\sum_h \sum_k c_{hk}n'_{hk} \leq (c_{ij} - c_{ij-1})n_{ij}(C) + \sum_h c_{hk(h)}N_h = C$$

so that

(22) $$n_{ij}(C) \geq \sum_h \sum_k (c_{hk} n'_{hk} - c_{hk(h)} N_h)(c_{ij} - c_{ij-1})^{-1}.$$

Consider the difference

$$Q(C) - Q = (q_{ij} - q_{ij-1})n_{ij}(C) + \sum_h q_{hk(h)} N_h - \sum_h \sum_k q_{hk} n'_{hk} .$$

Substituting for $n_{ij}(C)$ from (22) on the right-hand side of this equality gives

$$Q(C) - Q \geq R_{ij}^{-1} \sum_h \sum_k (c_{hk} n'_{hk} - c_{hk(h)} N_h) + \sum_h \sum_k (q_{hk} N_h - q_{hk} n'_{hk}) =$$

(23) $$R_{ij}^{-1} \sum_h \sum_k [(c_{hk} - R_{ij} q_{hk})n'_{hk} - (c_{hk(h)} - R_{ij} q_{hk(h)})N_h)] .$$

Now each term $- (c_{hk(h)} - R_{ij} q_{hk(h)})$ in (23) is non-negative. This is so if $R_{h2} > R_{ij}$ because in that case $hk(h) = h1$ and $c_{hk(h)} = q_{hk(h)} = 0$, and otherwise

$$c_{hk(h)} - R_{ij} q_{hk(h)} = q_{hk(h)} \left[\frac{c_{hk(h)}}{q_{hk(h)}} - R_{ij} \right] \leq q_{hk(h)}(R_{hk(h)} - R_{ij}) \leq 0,$$

where the inequality

$$\frac{c_{hk(h)}}{q_{hk(h)}} \leq R_{hk(h)}$$

follows from the ACE-ratio Corollary 3.2 and $R_{hk(h)} - R_{ij} \leq 0$ by hypothesis. Accordingly, replace N_h in (23) with $n'_{hk} \leq N_h$. Then the difference $Q(C) - Q$ is

(24) $$Q(C) - Q \geq R_{ij}^{-1} \sum_h \sum_k [(c_{hk} - c_{hk(h)}) - (q_{hk} - q_{hk(h)})]n'_{hk} =$$

$$R_{ij}^{-1} \sum_h \sum_k \left[\frac{c_{hk} - c_{hk(h)}}{q_{hk} - q_{hk(h)}} - R_{ij} \right](q_{hk} - q_{hk(h)})n'_{hk} .$$

Since $n'_{hk} \geq 0$, it remains to be shown in (24) that every term

$$\left[\frac{c_{hk} - c_{hk(h)}}{q_{hk} - q_{hk(h)}} - R_{ij} \right](q_{hk} - q_{hk(h)}) \geq 0.$$

Hence suppose first that $q_{hk} - q_{hk(h)} > 0$. Then

$$\frac{c_{hk} - c_{hk(h)}}{q_{hk} - q_{hk(h)}} > R_{ij}$$

because

$$\frac{c_{hk} - c_{hk(h)}}{q_{hk} - q_{hk(h)}} \geq \frac{c_{hk(h)+1} - c_{hk(h)}}{q_{hk(h)+1} - q_{hk(h)}} > \frac{c_{hk(h)} - c_{hk(h)-1}}{q_{hk(h)} - q_{hk(h)-1}}$$

by (5) of Lemma 2 and the ordering property of ICE ratios in a nondominated treatment set, and

$$\frac{c_{hk(h)} - c_{hk(h)-1}}{q_{hk(h)} - q_{hk(h)-1}} = R_{hk(h)} = \max_k \{R_{hk} \leq R_{ij}\}.$$

Next, suppose that $q_{hk} - q_{hk(h)} < 0$. In that event,

$$\frac{c_{hk} - c_{hk(h)}}{q_{hk} - q_{hk(h)}} < R_{ij}$$

because

$$\frac{c_{hk(h)} - c_{hk}}{q_{hk(h)} - q_{hk}} \leq \frac{c_{hk(h)} - c_{hk(h)-1}}{q_{hk(h)} - q_{hk(h)-1}} = R_{hk(h)}$$

by (4) of Lemma 2, and $R_{hk(h)} \leq R_{ij}$ by definition. Thus the product

$$\left[\frac{c_{hk} - c_{hk(h)}}{q_{hk} - q_{hk(h)}} - R_{ij}\right](q_{hk} - q_{hk(h)}) \geq 0$$

for every h, k, and k(h), the right-hand side of (24) is non-negative, and $Q(C) - Q \geq 0$. The global patient assignment asserted by (18)-(20) is therefore optimal, and the proof is now complete.

Several points are worth making regarding the proposition and its proof. First, it may seem that the proposition could be simplified somewhat by replacing the rank numbers of ICE ratios with the ICE ratios themselves, but this is not so because $\rho_{hk} < \rho_{ij}$ does not necessarily imply $R_{hk} < R_{ij}$. For example, suppose $R_{fp} = R_{gm} = R_{ij}$ for three different illnesses f, g, and i. The three ratios can be ranked in any order, but suppose $\rho_{gm} < \rho_{ij} < \rho_{fp}$ and that C is in $(C^{t-1}, C^t]$. Then by the proposition $n_{ij}(C)$ and $n_{ij-1}(C)$ are given by (18), and by (20) $n_{gm}(C) = N_g$ and $n_{fp}(C) = 0$ since $n_{fp-1}(C) = N_f$. However, if the rank numbers are replaced by ICE ratios so that from the second line of (19) hk(h) is such that

$$R_{hk(h)} = \max_{hk} \{R_{hk} \leq R_{ij}\},$$

then $n_{fp}(C) = N_f$ and $n_{fp-1}(C) = 0$. And because $c_{fp} > c_{fp-1}$, not only is this last solution non-optimal but it forces a violation of the total cost constraint as well.

It is important to note that the optimal total quantity of health benefits is unique. In particular,

Corollary 8. If there are groups of ICE ratios having equal values, the ratios can be ordered in any way within the groups without changing the optimal total quantity of health benefits.

Proof: Suppose $R_{hk} = R_{gm}$ for any two treatments hk $\neq$ gm. Suppose further that there are two prioritized orderings of all ICE ratios that are the same except for the rankings of R_{hk} and R_{gm}. Then however R_{hk} andf R_{gm} are ranked, the health care agency obtains an optimal global patient assignment from each of the prioritized orderings of all ICE ratios. If the assignments are the same the claim is trivial, so assume they are not. But if $\rho_{hk} < \rho_{gm}$, the optimality of the assignment that results implies that it produces at least as large a total quantity of health benefits as any other global assignment, and the same is true for the optimal global assignment if $\rho_{hk} > \rho_{gm}$. Thus even though the optimal global assignments may differ, the two optimal total quantiies of health benefits must be equal.

The optimal assignment policy prioritizes treatments and does this by ordering the ICE ratios defined on them—by the values of their marginal costs. As total cost C increases, the endpoints of the budget intervals that contain C increase, and therefore the ICE ratios R_{ij} associated with these intervals tend to increase as well. (In general the identity of illness i changes as C increases.) In turn, by (19) and (20) the maximum ICE ratio $R_{hk(h)} \leq R_{ij}$ also increases or does not decrease. Hence as the agency's budget increases the optimal global patient assignment changes so that treatments having progressively higher marginal costs of health benefits are provided to or insured for patients.

The salient properties of the optimal total quantity of health benefits

Q(C) were listed in the preceding section, and proofs of most of these properties can be obtained easily from (18)-(20). For instance, given that the cost constraint is everywhere binding on $[0,C^T]$:

(i) Q(C) is continuous and piecewise linear on $[0,C^T]$. This result follows immediately from (18)-(20) and (21) because for C in $(C^{t-1}, C^t]$ and R_{ij},

$$(25) \qquad Q(C) = (q_{ij} - q_{ij-1})n_{ij}(C) + \sum_h q_{hk(h)}N_h = \frac{C}{R_{ij}} + \left[Q(C^{t-1}) - \frac{C^{t-1}}{R_{ij}} \right].$$

Thus Q(C) is linear in $(C^{t-1}, C^t]$ with slope $1/R_{ij}$. By (25) Q(C) is continuous on the right at each budget point C^{t-1} for $t \geq 1$ since it is obvious that $Q(C) \rightarrow Q(C^{t-1})$ as $C \rightarrow C^{t-1}$. But also by (25) Q(C) is continuous on the left at C^t inasmuch as

$$Q(C) = (q_{ij} - q_{ij-1})n_{ij}(C) + \sum_h q_{hk(h)}N_h = (q_{ij} - q_{ij-1})n_{ij}(C) +$$

$$q_{ij-1}N_i + \sum_{h \neq i} q_{hk(h)}N_h$$

and by (18) $n_{ij}(C) \rightarrow N_i$ as $C \rightarrow C^t$. Thus as $C \rightarrow C^t$,

$$Q(C) \rightarrow (q_{ij}N_i - q_{ij-1}N_i + q_{ij-1}N_i + \sum_{h \neq i} q_{hk(h)}N_h) = \sum_h q_{hk(h)}N_h = Q(C^t).$$

Accordingly, Q(C) is continuous everywhere on $[0,C^T]$.

(ii) Q(C) is monotone strictly increasing on $[0,C^T]$. This property of Q(C) results from continuity and the fact that all of the linear segments of Q(C) are positively sloped.

(iii) The partial derivative

$$\frac{\partial Q(C)}{\partial C}$$

exists and is continuous everywhere on $[0,C^T]$ except possibly at one or more of the budget points C^t. From (24)

$$\frac{\partial Q(C)}{\partial C} = \frac{1}{R_{ij}}$$

at all C in (C^{t-1}, C^t), and

$$\lim_{C \to C^{t-1}} \left[\frac{Q(C) - Q(C^{t-1})}{C - C^{t-1}} \right] =$$

$$\lim_{C \to C^{t-1}} \left\{ \left[\frac{C}{R_{ij}} + Q(C^{t-1}) - \frac{C^{t-1}}{R_{ij}} - Q(C^{t-1}) \right] (C - C^{t-1})^{-1} \right\} =$$

$$\lim_{C \to C^{t-1}} \frac{1}{R_{ij}} = \frac{1}{R_{ij}}.$$

Similarly,

$$\lim_{C \to C^t} \left[\frac{Q(C^t) - Q(C)}{C^t - C} \right] =$$

$$\lim_{C \to C^t} \left\{ \left[\frac{(C^t - C^{t-1})}{R_{ij}} + Q(C^{t-1}) - \frac{(C - C^{t-1})}{R_{ij}} - Q(C^{t-1}) \right] (C - C^{t-1})^{-1} \right\} = \frac{1}{R_{ij}}$$

Thus

$$\frac{\partial Q(C)}{\partial C}$$

exists as a right-hand partial derivative at C^{t-1} and as a left hand partial derivative at C^t. But it has the same properties as these in the bordering budget intervals $(C^{t-2}, C^{t-1}]$ and $(C^t, C^{t+1}]$, which is to say that

$$\frac{\partial Q(C)}{\partial C} = \begin{cases} 1/R_{gm} \text{ in } (C^{t-2}, C^{t-1}] \\ 1/R_{ij} \text{ in } (C^{t-1}, C^t] \\ 1/R_{hk} \text{ in } (C^t, C^{t+1}] \end{cases}$$

for some ICE ratios R_{gm} and R_{hk}. Unless $R_{gm} = R_{ij} = R_{hk}$,

$$\frac{\partial Q(C)}{\partial C}$$

is discontinuous at C^{t-1} and C^t, and, more generally, it is not necessarily continuous at any budget points in $[0, C^T]$.

(iv) $Q(C)$ is concave on $[0, C^T]$. The concavity of $Q(C)$ is evident from continuity and the result that the slopes $1/R_{ij}$ of the segments of $Q(C)$ are nonincreasing in C. However, a formal proof is given in Appendix 3.2 at the end of the chapter.

(v) Maximum total health benefits $Q(C)$ is unique at each C in $[0, C^T]$. This claim follows from (iv).

(vi) The marginal cost of health benefits at the optimum,

$$\frac{\partial C(Q)}{\partial Q} = \frac{1}{\frac{\partial Q(C)}{\partial C}}$$

is a nondecreasing function of Q. Let $(C^{s-1}, C^s]$ and $(C^{t-1}, C^t]$ be adjacent budget intervals associated with ICE ratios R_{hk} and R_{ij} and such that $C^s = C^{t-1}$. Then if C^1 is in $(C^{s-1}, C^s]$ and C^2 is in $(C^{t-1}, C^t]$, $C^1 < C^2$. From

(25) $$\frac{\partial Q(C)}{\partial C} = \frac{1}{R_{hk}}$$

for all C^1 in $(C^{s-1}, C^s]$ and $= 1/R_{ij}$ for all C^2 in $(C^{t-1}, C^t]$. But $R_{hk} \leq R_{ij}$ by the ordering property of all ICE ratios so that

$$\frac{\partial Q(C)}{\partial C}$$

is monotone nonincreasing in C. Hence the inverse function

$$\frac{\partial C(Q)}{\partial Q}$$

is monotone nondecreasing in Q.

(vii) At the optimum the (global) marginal cost of health benefits is R_{ij}. To see that consider the inverse function $Q^{-1}(C) = C(Q)$. Assume C is in $(C^{t-1}, C^t]$ and $\rho^t = R_{ij}$. Since by (18)-(20),

$$Q(C) = (q_{ij} - q_{ij-1})n_{ij}(C) + \sum_h q_{hk(h)}N_h = (q_{ij} - q_{ij-1})n_{ij}(C) + Q(C^{t-1})$$

and

$$n_{ij}(C) = \frac{C - C^{t-1}}{c_{ij} - c_{ij-1}},$$

one has $Q(C) = (C - C^t) R_{ij}^{-1} + Q(C^{t-1})$ at the optimum. Hence

$$C = R_{ij}Q + C^{t-1} - R_{ij}Q^{t-1} \text{ and } \frac{\partial C}{\partial Q} = R_{ij}$$

at the optimum.

Remark 8. By (vii) R_{ij} is the largest of all the marginal costs of health benefits at the optimum. Hence $R_{ij} = 1/\lambda(C)$ is the GM health care agency's cutoff point. In practice R_{ij} is the largest ICE ratio defined on any pair of treatments in the agency's health care system—i.e. it is the largest ICE ratio defined on any treatments hk and hk-1 such that $c_{hk} > c_{hk-1}, q_{hk} >$

q_{hk-1}, and a positive number of patients is assigned to hk. The result is used in the derivation of the single-treatment decision rules for the GM agency model.

Because the single-treatment analyst is not likely to know which two treatments ij and ij-1 define the GM agency's cutoff point, hereafter it will usually be denoted R(C) rather than R_{ij}. The R_{ij} notation will be reserved for proofs of some of the propositions that remain.

3.4 The Prioritizing Procedure: Two Examples

As has been remarked, the decision rules (18)-(20) are straightforward and easily applied. To see this is so consider the example of a hypothetical health care agency whose patient community suffers from three illnesses numbered 1-3. The sizes of the ill populations are 2,000, 3,000, and 4,000 patients respectively. Initially there are four active treatments each for illnesses 1 and 2 and three for illness 3. The costs and health benefits of all eleven active and three no-action treatments are shown in Table 3.1. Assume the agency's budget is $40 million, and that its task is to find an optimal global patient assignment at this total treatment cost.

In order to follow the prioritizing procedure described in the last section the agency or its analyst should take these steps.

1. Remove the dominated treatments, if there are any, from the initial treatment set. In Table 3.1 the initial sets of treatments for all three illnesses are ordered and indexed so that treatment costs are monotone nondecreasing in the treatment indexes. By the methods set out in Chapter 2 it is apparent that the initial treatment 13 for illness 1 is strictly strongly dominated by treatment 12, and that the initial treatment 23 for illness 2 is weakly dominated by treatments 22 and 24. The treatments for illness 3 are such that treatment costs, treatment health benefits, and the ICE ratios measured on adjacent treatments in the ordered set all strictly

increase in the treatment index. Hence by Proposition 5 the initial treatment set for illness 3 contains no dominated treatments. Treatments 13 and 23 and only these treatments are then removed from the initial treatment set.

Table 3.1

Example of Global CEA by Prioritization:

Cost and Health Benefit Data for Treatments of Three Illnesses

Illness & Treatment Hk	Cost Per Patient $c_{hk}(\$)$	Health Benefits Per Patient (q_{hk})	ICE Ratio R_{hk} ($/Benefit)	Population Size
11	0	0	--	$N_1 = 2,000$
12	1,000	0.3	3,333	
13	1,750	0.25	--	
14	3,200	0.65	3,625	
15	7,000	1.05	9,500	
21	0	0	--	$N_2 = 3,000$
22	150	0.2	750	
23	800	0.3	6,500	
24	1,800	0.5	5,000	
25	3,100	0.7	6,500	
31	0	0	--	$N_3 = 4,000$
32	3,000	1.0	3,000	
33	8,000	1.5	10,000	
34	16,000	2.0	16,000	

2. Separately for each illness reorder and reindex the remaining treatments so that treatment costs and health benefits strictly increase in the (new) treatment index. Recompute the ICE ratios measured on adjacent treatments in each of the ordered sets. The three treatment sets produced by these operations are shown in Table 3.2. The ordered

treatment sets for all three illnesses are now such that treatment costs, treatment health benefits, and ICE ratios strictly increase in the respective treatment indexes. Therefore again by Proposition 5 the three treatment sets now contain only nondominated treatments. The total number of nondominated active treatments is T = 9.

Table 3.2
Example of Global CEA by Prioritization:
Cost and Health Benefit Data for Treatments of Three Ilnesses
After Dominated Treatments Are Deleted

Illness & Treatment hk	Cost Per Patient $c_{hk}(\$)$	Health Benefits Per Patient (q_{hk})	ICE Ratio R_{hk} (\$/Benefit)	Population Size
11	0	0	--	$N_1 = 2,000$
12	1,000	0.3	3,333	
13	3,200	0.65	6,286	
14	7,000	1.05	9,500	
21	0	0	--	$N_2 = 3,000$
22	150	0.2	750	
23	1,800	0.5	5,500	
24	3,100	0.7	6,500	
31	0	0	--	$N_3 = 4,000$
32	3,000	1.0	3,000	
33	8,000	1.5	10,000	
34	16,000	2.0	16,000	

3. Order the T = 9 ICE ratios from smallest to largest. Assign the rank number 1 to the smallest ratio and the rank number 9 to the largest. The second column of Table 3.3 displays the ranked ICE ratios. The third column identifies the costlier of the two treatments on which the ratios are measured.

4. Compute the values of the budget points C^1, C^2,..., C^9 using (17). These are shown in the fourth column of Table 3.3. For instance, in millions of dollars $C^7 = C^6 + (c_{14} - c_{13})N_1 = 27.7 + [(7,000-3,200) \times 2,000]10^{-6} = 35.3$. Each pair of budget points then generates a budget interval such as $(C^6, C^7] = (27.7, 35.3]$ valued in millions of dollars.

Table 3.3
Example of Global CEA by Prioritization:
The Optimal Treatment Priorities

t	R_{hk} ($/Benefit)	Treat-ment hk	Budget Points $C^t = C^{t-1} + (c_{hk} - c_{hk-1})N_h$ ($ millions)	Optimal Treatment Set at C = C^t	Treatment Enters Optimal Treatment Set at C^{t-1}	Treatment Exits Optimal Treatment Set at C^t
0	--	--	0	11,21,31	--	
1	750	22	0.45	11,22,31	22	21
2	3,000	32	12.45	11,22,32	32	31
3	3,333	12	14.45	12,22,32	12	11
4	5,500	23	19.40	12,23,32	23	22
5	6,286	13	23.80	13,23,32	13	12
6	6,500	24	27.70	13,24,32	24	23
7	9,500	14	35.30	14,24,32	14	13
8	10,000	33	55.30	14,24,33	33	32
9	16,000	34	87.30	14,24,34	34	33

The *set of optimal treatments*—the treatments to which positive numbers of patients are optimally assigned—at each C^t is shown in column 5 of Table 3.3. Although they are not necessary for finding optimal global assignments, the treatments entering and exiting the optimal treatment set at each budget point are presented in the sixth and seventh columns of the table.

To obtain the optimal global patient assignment at the total cost of $40 million, first find the budget interval that contains this total cost and then apply (18)-(20). In this example total cost is a point in the budget interval $(C^7, C^8]$, or in millions of dollars, $35.30 < 40 \le 55.30$. Thus ij = 33, ij-1 = 32, and with treatment costs in dollars and total costs in millions of dollars, the optimal global patient assignment is

$$n_{33}(C) = (C - C^7)/(c_{33} - c_{32}) = 1,000,000 \times (40 -$$
$$35.3)/(8,000 - 3,000) = 940$$
$$n_{32}(C) = N_3 - n_{33}(C) = 4,000 - 940 = 3,060$$
$$n_{24}(C) = N_2 = 3,000$$
$$n_{14}(C) = N_1 = 2,000$$

all other $n_{hk}(C) = 0$.

The total health benefit produced by the assignment is $940 \times 1.5 + 3,060 \times 1.0 + 3,000 \times 0.7 + 2,000 \times 1.05 = 8,670$ units. Treatments 14, 24, 32, and 33 are—and are the only— members of *the optimal treatment* set at $C = \$40$ million, and at this total cost they are—and are the only—absolutely cost-effective treatments for illness 1, 2 and 3. Also observe that the health care system's cutoff point at $C = \$40$ million—the largest ICE ratio R_{ij} such that $n_{ij}(C) > 0$—is $R_{33} = \$10,000$ per unit of health benefits. It has been said that Q(C) is unique but that the optimal global assignment need not be, and a second example demonstrates that possibility.

For example, assume there exists a fifth treatment 25 for illness 2, that its unit cost is $4,100, and that it produces 0.8 units of health benefits per patient. Then

$$R_{25} = \frac{c_{25} - c_{24}}{q_{25} - q_{24}} = \$10,000 \text{ per unit of health benefits}$$

and $R_{25} = R_{33}$. Hence R_{25} can be given a higher or lower rank than R_{33} in the ordered set of all ICE ratios and the optimal total volume of health benefits is the same. Suppose first that R_{25} is given the next lower rank than R_{33}. Then the first three columns of Table 3.3 must be revised slightly and the revisions are shown in the first three columns of Table 3.4. Now $40 million is a point in the budget interval $(C^8, C^9]$ and in millions of dollars $38.30 < 40 \leq 55.30$. Thus $ij = 33$, $ij-1 = 32$, and, again with treatment costs in dollars and total costs in millions, the new optimal global assignment is

$$n_{33}(C) = (C - C^8)/(c_{34} - c_{33}) = 1,000,000 \times (40 -$$
$$38.3)/(16,000 - 8,000) = 340$$
$$n_{32}(C) = 4,000 - n_{33}(C) = 3,660$$
$$n_{14}(C) = 2,000$$
$$n_{25}(C) = 3,000$$
all other $n_{hk}(C) = 0$.

The total health benefit produced by this new global patient assignment $Q(C) = 340 \times 1.5 + 3,660 \times 1.0 + 2,000 \times 1.05 + 3,000 \times 0.8 = 8,670$ units.

Now let R_{25} be given the next higher rank than R_{33}. The prioritized global treatment set for this ranking of R_{25} and R_{33} is shown in Table 3.5. As it is for the prioritized treatment set presented in Table 3.3, the total cost $40 million is a point in the budget interval $(C^7, C^8]$. The optimal global assignment at $40 million is therefore the same as the optimal assignment obtained from the Table 3.3 figures, and the optimal total quantity of health benefits is the same as well, 8,670 units. Here the optimal global assignments differ depending on the rankings of R_{33} and R_{25} but the optimal total quantity of health benefits does not.

In the example it happens that $10,000 per unit of health beneifits is the health care system's cutoff point and that the cutoff point is defined by either R_{33} or R_{25} depending on how the two ratios are ranked, but this is not essential for illustrating the ranking property that gives the equality of the optimal quantities of health benefits. Assume that total treatment cost is $80 million so that the cutoff point is $16,000 per unit of health benefits and defined by treatments 34 and 33. Then by inspection of Tables 3.4 and 3.5 it is evident that the optimal global patient assignment is the same whether R_{25} is given the next higher or next lower rank than R_{33}. The optimal global assignment for each ranking is

$$n_{34}(C) = (C - C^9)/(c_{34} - c_{33}) =$$
$$1,000,000 \times (80 - 58.3)/(16,000 - 8,000) = 2,712.5$$
$$n_{33}(C) = 4,000 - n_{34}(C) = 1,287.5$$

Table 3.4
Example of Global CEA by Prioritization:
The Revised Optimal Treatment Priorities

t	R_{hk} ($/Benefit)	Treat-ment hk	Budget Points $C^t = C^{t-1} + (c_{hk}-c_{hk-1})N_h$ ($ millions)	Optimal Treatment Set at C = C^t	Treatment Enters Optimal Treatment Set at C^{t-1}	Treatment Exits Optimal Treatment Set at C^t
0	--	--	0	11,21,31	--	
1	750	22	0.45	11,22,31	22	21
2	3,000	32	12.45	11,22,32	32	31
3	3,333	12	14.45	12,22,32	12	11
4	5,500	23	19.40	12,23,32	23	22
5	6,286	13	23.80	13,23,32	13	12
6	6,500	24	27.70	13,24,32	24	23
7	9,500	14	35.30	14,24,32	14	13
8	10,000	25	38.30	14,25,32	25	24
9	10,000	33	58.30	14,25,33	33	32
10	16,000	34	90.30	14,25,34	34	33

Table 3.5
Example of Global CEA by Prioritization:
The Second Revision of Optimal Treatment Priorities

t	R_{hk} ($/Benefit)	Treat-ment hk	Budget Points $C^t = C^{t-1} + (c_{hk}-c_{hk-1})N_h$ ($ millions)	Optimal Treatment Set at C = C^t	Treatment Enters Optimal Treatment Set at C^{t-1}	Treatment Exits Optimal Treatment Set at C^t
0	--	--	0	11,21,31	--	
1	750	22	0.45	11,22,31	22	21
2	3,000	32	12.45	11,22,32	32	31
3	3,333	12	14.45	12,22,32	12	11
4	5,500	23	19.40	12,23,32	23	22
5	6,286	13	23.80	13,23,32	13	12
6	6,500	24	27.70	13,24,32	24	23
7	9,500	14	35.30	14,24,32	14	13
8	10,000	33	55.30	14,24,33	33	32
9	10,000	25	58.30	14,25,33	25	24
10	16,000	34	90.30	14,25,34	34	33

$n_{25}(C) = 3,000$

all other $n_{hk}(C) = 0$.

Other examples of the prioritization technique are given in Chapter 6. There they are used to verify the conclusions of examples of single-treatment CEA for the GM agency model.

3.5 Global Maximization and Single-Treatment Cost-Effectiveness Analysis

The next chapter presents the single-treatment decision rules for absolute cost-effectiveness when the health care agency is a global maximizer. Some of the rules follow directly from Proposition 8, but it is useful here to give a second proposition from which they can also be derived. Both the proposition and the derivations of the rules in Chapter 4 address the positioning of budget intervals after a new nondominated treatment $h\hat{k}$ has been added to the set of all treatments for illness h. The optimality of the health care agency's initial global assignment given by Proposition 8 hinges on the location of C in the budget interval $(C^{t-1}, C^t]$. But when $h\hat{k}$ enters the treatment set for h it creates one or two new ICE ratios defined on treatments in the new ordered set of all treatments. These are $R_{h\hat{k}}$ defined on $h\hat{k}$ and the next costliest, most health-benefit productive treatment in the new ordered set, and, if there is a treatment $h\hat{k} + 1$, $R_{h\hat{k}+1}$ defined on $h\hat{k}$ and the next costliest, most health-benefit productive treatment in the set. In turn, $R_{h\hat{k}}$ and $R_{h\hat{k}+1}$ create one or two new budget intervals that are added to the ordered set of all budget intervals. Depending on how they are positioned in the set of all budget intervals, these new intervals can displace the endpoints of the budget interval associated with R_{ij} so that they are larger or smaller than those of $(C^{t-1}, C^t]$. Entering $h\hat{k}$ into the treatment set for h may also cause the removal of some ICE ratios including R_{ij} from the ordered set of all ICE ratios, with the consequence that one or more of the initial budget intervals are also removed from the ordered set of all budget intervals.

Thus C may no longer be in $(C^{t-1}, C^t]$, but whether it is or is not, in general there can be a new optimal global patient assignment. The decision rules of Chapter 4 give necessary and sufficient conditions for $h\hat{k}$ to be a member of the new optimal treatment set—for $h\hat{k}$ to be absolutely cost-effective for h—and they are proved by determining the effect on the initial ordered set of all budget intervals of entering $h\hat{k}$ into the treatment set for h. Proposition 8 gives a means for making that determination.

Proposition 9. Let $(C^{s-1}, C^s]$ be the budget interval associated with $R_{h\hat{k}}$ and treatment $h\hat{k}$. If there is a treatment $h\hat{k}+1$, let $(C^{s'-1}, C^{s'}]$ be the budget interval associated with $R_{h\hat{k}+1}$ and treatment $h\hat{k}+1$. Then if there is

(i) a treatment $h\hat{k}+1$, $h\hat{k}$ is optimal for illness h at all C such that $C^{s-1} < C < C^{s'}$.

(ii) no treatment $h\hat{k}+1$, $h\hat{k}$ is optimal for illness h at all $C > C^{s-1}$.

Proof of (i): $h\hat{k}$ is optimal for h at all C in $(C^{s-1}, C^s]$ by (18) of Proposition 8 with $h\hat{k}$ replacing ij. Also by (18) of Proposition 8, $h\hat{k}$ and $h\hat{k}+1$ are both optimal for h at all C in $(C^{s'-1}, C^{s'}]$, with $h\hat{k}+1$ replacing ij and $h\hat{k}$ replacing ij-1, except at $C^{s'}$ since $n_{hk}(C^{s'}) = 0$. Next, $R_{h\hat{k}} < R_{h\hat{k}+1}$ implies $\rho_{h\hat{k}} < \rho_{h\hat{k}+1}$. Hence by the one-to-one orderings of ICE-ratios and budget intervals, $C^s \le C^{s'-1}$. If $C^s = C^{s'-1}$ the validity of (i) is immediate, so suppose $C^s < C^{s'-1}$. In that case $h\hat{k}$ replaces ij in (18) of Proposition 9 and

$$\rho_{h\hat{k}} = \max_m \{\rho_{hm} < \rho_{h\hat{k}}\}$$

at all C such that $C^s < C < C^{s'-1}$. Treatment $h\hat{k}$ is optimal at all such C by (19) and (20) of Proposition 8, and therefore $h\hat{k}$ is optimal at all C in the intervals $(C^{s-1}, C^s]$, $(C^s, C^{s'-1}]$, and $(C^{s'-1}, C^{s'}]$. This result completes the proof of (i).

Proof of (ii): Again $h\hat{k}$ is optimal at all C in $(C^{s-1}, C^s]$ by Proposition 8 with $h\hat{k}$ replacing ij. Then if $C > C^s$, C is in a budget interval $(C^{t-1}, C^t]$

where $C^s < C^{t-1}$ and the interval is associated with the ICE-ratio rank ρ_{ij}. Moreover, by the one-to-one orderings of budget intervals and ICE-ratio ranks, $\rho_{h\hat{k}} < \rho_{ij}$. Because there is no $h\hat{k}+1$, it follows that

$$\rho_{h\hat{k}} = \max_m \{\rho_{hm} < \rho_{h\hat{k}}\},$$

and $h\hat{k}$ is optimal for h by (19) and (20) of Proposition 8. Thus $h\hat{k}$ is optimal at all C in $(C^{s-1}, C^s]$ and in all C in every budget interval $(C^{t-1}, C^t]$ for all t = s+1, s+2,..., T, and the proof of (ii) is complete
.

Appendix 3. Proof of the Concavity of Q(C)

A function f(x) defined on a one- or multidimensional interval D is concave (convex) if for any $\underline{x}$ and $\underline{x}$ in D and all numbers δ such that $0 \le \delta \le 1$, $f[\delta\underline{x} + (1-\delta)\underline{x}] \ge (\le) \delta f(\underline{x}) + (1-\delta)f(\underline{x})$. Obviously, all linear functions are both concave and convex. Thus total costs

$$\sum_h \sum_k c_{hk} n_{hk} \text{ and total health benefits } \sum_h \sum_k q_{hk} n_{hk}$$

are both concave and convex in the n_{hk}.

Proposition. Q(C) is concave on $[0, C^T]$.

Proof: The proof given here is a special case of a more general proof by Dixit [1976, p. 51]. What must be shown is that for any two total costs $\underline{C}$ and $\underline{C}$ in $[0, C^T]$ and for any δ, $0 \le \delta \le 1$,

(26) $\qquad\qquad Q[\delta\underline{C} + (1-\delta)\underline{C}] \ge \delta Q(\underline{C}) + (1-\delta)Q(\underline{C})$.

Let

$$Q(n_{hk}) = \sum_h \sum_k q_{hk} n_{hk} \; .$$

Then there are optimal global assignments $(\underline{n}_{hk})$ and $(\underline{n}_{hk})$ such that $Q(\underline{n}_{hk}) = Q(\underline{C})$ and $Q(\underline{n}_{hk}) = Q(\underline{C})$. Let

$$C(n_{hk}) = \sum_h \sum_k c_{hk} n_{hk} \; .$$

Accordingly, $\underline{C} = C(\underline{n}_{hk})$, $\underline{C} = C(\underline{n}_{hk})$, and because $C(n_{hk})$ is convex in the n_{hk},

$$C[\delta\underline{n}_{hk} + (1-\delta)\underline{n}_{hk}] \le \delta C(\underline{n}_{hk}) + (i-\delta)C(\underline{n}_{hk}) = \delta\underline{C} + (1-\delta)\underline{C}.$$

That is, the cost of the new global assignment $(\delta \underline{n}_{hk} + (1-\delta)\underline{n}_{hk})$ is no greater than the constraint $\delta \underline{C} + (1-\delta)\underline{C}$. Next, and since $Q(\underline{n}_{hk})$ is concave in the n_{hk}, the same global assignment and same δ give

$$Q[\delta \underline{n}_{hk} + (1-\delta)\underline{n}_{hk}] \geq \delta Q(\underline{n}_{hk}) + (i-\delta)Q(\underline{n}_{hk}) = \delta Q(\underline{C}) + (1-\delta)Q(\underline{C}).$$

Therefore, there exists at least one global assignment $(\delta \underline{n}_{hk} + (1-\delta)\underline{n}_{hk})$, that costs no more than $\delta \underline{C} + (1-\delta)\underline{C}$ and that produces at least as large a total health benefit as $\delta Q(\underline{C}) + (1-\delta)Q(\underline{C})$. This result is already sufficient to establish (26), but there may also be other global assignments that cost no more $\delta \underline{C} + (1-\delta)\underline{C}$ and that produce an even larger volume of health benefits than $Q[\delta \underline{n}_{hk} + (1-\delta)\underline{n}_{hk}]$. Thus in that event,

$$Q[\delta \underline{C} + (1-\delta)\underline{C}] > \delta Q(\underline{n}_{hk}) + (i-\delta)Q(\underline{n}_{hk}) = \delta Q(\underline{C}) + (1-\delta)Q(\underline{C}).$$

The inequality establishes (26) and the proof is now complete.

References

Blumstein JF. The Oregon experiment: The role of cost-benefit analysis in the allocation of Medicaid funds. Social Science and Medicine 1997; 45: 545-554.

Dantzig GB. Linear Programming and Extensions. Princeton, NJ: Princeton University Press, 1963.

Dantzig GB, Thapa MN. Linear Programming. I: Introduction. New York: Springer-Verlag, 1997.

Dorfman R, Samuelson PA, Solow RM. Linear Programming and Economic Analysis. New York: McGraw-Hill Book Company. 1958.

Dixit AK. Optimization in Economic Theory. London: Oxford University Press, 1976.

Eddy DM. Oregon's methods? Did cost-effectiveness analysis fail? JAMA 1991; 266: 2135-2141.

Fox DM, Leichter HM. State model: Oregon. Health Affairs 1993; 12: 66-70.

Hadorn DC. Setting health care priorities in Oregon. Cost-effectiveness analysis meets the rule of rescue. JAMA 1991; 265: 2218-2225.

Johansson P-O. An Introduction to Modern Welfare Economics. Cambridge, UK: Cambridge University Press, 1991.

Kaplan RM. Value judgment in the Oregon Medicaid experiment.

Medical Care 1994; 32: 975-988.

Kaplan RM, Anderson JP. The General Health Policy Model: an integrated approach. In: Spiker B. (ed.) Quality of Life Assessments in Clinical trials. New York: Raven Press, 1990.

Kaplan RM, Anderson JP. A general health policy model: update and applications. Health Services Research 1988; 23: 203-235.

Karlsson G, Johannesson M. The decision rules of cost-effectiveness analysis. Pharmacoeconomics 1996; 9: 113-120.

Kitzhaber JA. Prioritizing health services in an era of limits: the Oregon experience. BMJ 1993; 307: 373-377.

Laska EM, Meisner M, Siegel C, Stinnett AA. Ratio-based and net benefit-based approaches to health care resource allocation: proofs of optimality and equivalence. Health Economics 1999; 8: 171-174.

Rudin W. Principles of Mathematical Analysis (3rd ed.). New York: McGraw-Hill, 1976.

Stinnett AA, Paltiel AD. Mathematical programming for the efficient allocation of health care resources. Journal of Health Economics 1996; 15: 641-653.

Takayama A. Analytical Methods in Economics. Ann Arbor: University of Michigan Press, 1993.

Torrance GW, Thomas WH, Sackett DL. A utility maximization model for evaluation of health care programs. Health Services Research 1972; 7: 118-133.

Varian HR. Microeconomic Analysis (3rd ed.). New York: WW Norton & Co., 1992.

Weiner JM. Oregon's plan for health care rationing. The Brookings Review 1992;10: 26-31.

Weinstein MC, Fineberg HV. Clinical Decision Analysis. Philadelphia: WB Saunders, 1980.

4 Deterministic Single-Treatment Cost-Effectiveness Analysis in the Global Maximizer Model: the Decision Rules

4.1 The Decision Problem in Single-treatment Cost-Effectiveness Analysis

The most common problem in conventional CEAs consists of deciding which of two treatments for a focal (particular) illness should be provided to or sanctioned for patients and is therefore a—or the—cost-effective treatment for the illness. Ordinarily one of the two treatments is new and the other is a current or standard treatment for the illness. Although the decision problem will be broadened in this and the following chapters to allow the agency to choose among two or more treatments for the illnesses, the convention will be maintained that the one to be tested is new. In the preceding chapter it was assumed that the health care agency is a global maximizer and that assumption will be maintained in this chapter as well. Two definitions of cost-effectiveness were given in Chapter 1: relative, which refers to the comparative costs and health benefits of two treatments for the focal illness, and absolute, which refers to comparative costs and health benefits of all treatments for the illness. The concept of relative cost-effectiveness is, however, irrelevant for the decision making of a GM agency. A new or any treatment is either optimal in the sense of (18)-(20) of Proposition 8 or it is not, and it can be cost-effective relative to some other treatment for the illness without being optimal or appropriate to provide or insure for patients. Accordingly, the definition of cost-effectiveness for the decision rules of single-treatment CEA with the GM theory is this.

Definition. A treatment is absolutely cost-effective (and should be provided to or insured for patients) if and only if it satisfies the optimality conditions (18)-(20) of Proposition 8.

Let $h\hat{k}$ be a new treatment for illness h. Then given total cost C, $h\hat{k}$ is absolutely cost-effective for h if the agency's optimal global patient assignment is such that a positive number of patients is assigned to $h\hat{k}$. It follows also that $h\hat{k}$ is cost-effective relative to every other treatment for h because for any global assignment in which $n_{h\hat{k}}$ = 0, it is always possible to switch patients from other treatments to $h\hat{k}$ and by that action increase or not reduce total health benefits without increasing total cost.

The information requirements for conducting single-treatment CEAs were stated in Chapter 1. They are the values or estimates of the values of the

- costs of all treatments for h, and
- health benefits of all treatments for h.

In addition the analyst must know the health care system's cutoff point or have some procedure for incorporating it into the CEA. Let R(C) be the GM agency's cutoff point. It was shown in Chapter 3 that R(C) is the marginal cost of producing health benefits

$$R_{ij} = \frac{c_{ij} - c_{ij-1}}{q_j - q_{ij-1}}$$

at the optimal global patient assignment. In (18)-(20) of Proposition 8 it is also shown that R_{ij} is the largest ICE ratio defined on treatments (on ij and ij-1) to which positive numbers of patients are assigned. If $R_{hk} > R_{ij}$, no patient is assigned to either hk or hk-1. *Empirically, the cutoff point should therefore be taken or estimated as the largest observed marginal cost of producing health benefits in the given health care system.* Any other empirical definition of R(C) is incompatible with the theoretical definition given by the GM model.

When a value or estimate of R(C) is either unavailable or untrustworthy, the simplest strategy is to make R(C) a parameter of the analysis. In that case the CEA can be performed so as to state that $h\hat{k}$ is or can be declared absolutely cost-effective if and only if R(C) is a point in a particular critical interval of values. The user of the CEA then decides whether or not R(C) is a point in this critical interval and *ipso facto* whether or not $h\hat{k}$ is absolutely cost-effective.

The single-treatment decision rules for absolute cost-effectiveness are simple ones, but proving their validity is unfortunately a somewhat laborious undertaking. The rules are derived here from Propositions 8 and 9. If the new treatment $h\hat{k}$ is dominated, it is not absolutely cost-effective and the CEA immediately terminates. But when a nondominated new treatment is added to the set of all treatments, it causes the creation of one or two new budget intervals and it can also cause the deletion of one or more of the initial budget intervals associated with treatments for h. To apply Propositions 8 and 9, the composition and ordering of the new set of all budget intervals must therefore be ascertained in order to discover which of these intervals now contains total cost C.

The principal methodological problem concerns the effect on the ordered set of all budget intervals when $h\hat{k}$ dominates at least one of the initial treatments for h. The problem is taken up in the next section.

4.2 Treatment Dominance and the Structure of New Treatment Sets

In the prioritization method for selecting an optimal global patient assignment all dominated treatments are first removed from the treatment set for every illness. So assume the initial (optimal) treatment set for the focal illness h contains no dominated treatments and assume further that the set is ordered so that treatment costs, treatment health benefits, and the ICE ratios defined on adjacent treatment pairs all strictly increase in the treatment index. The initial ordered set of treatments for h is {h1, h2, ..., hk,..., hK}. Now assume treatment $h\hat{k}$ is added to the initial treatment set and that it is not dominated by any of the other treatments for h. Then there are two issues to be considered. First, if $h\hat{k}$ dominates one or more of the initial treatments and these treatments are deleted, how is treatment set restructured and ordered by the deletions? Second, whether or not it dominates other treatments for h, how is $h\hat{k}$ placed in the new ordered set of treatments for h? These questions are of importance because the composition and order of the new treatment set for h determines the composition and order of the new set of all budget intervals when $h\hat{k}$ enters the treatment set. In turn, the configuration of the new set of budget intervals determines the agency's new optimal global assignment and whether or not $h\hat{k}$ is a member of the optimal treatment set. The two propositions presented in this section, Propositions 10 and 11, address the two structuring and ordering questions. The proof of Proposition 10 is lengthy on account of the number of different ways treatments can be dominated, and it is therefore divided and given in the following four parts.

Lemma 3. Assume a new treatment $h\hat{k}$ is added to the treatment set for h and assume it is not dominated. Then if $h\hat{k}$ strongly dominates an initial treatment hk for illness h but does not strongly or weakly dominate

(i) treatment hk+1, it does not strongly dominate any treatment hd such that $d > k+1$.

(ii) treatment hk-1, it does not strongly dominate any treatment hd such that $d < k+1$.

Proof of (i): If $h\hat{k}$ does not strongly dominate hk+1, either $c_{h\hat{k}} > c_{hk+1}$, $q_{h\hat{k}} > q_{hk+1}$ or $c_{h\hat{k}} < c_{hk+1}$, $q_{h\hat{k}} < q_{hk+1}$. The first pair of inequalities is impossible because then $c_{h\hat{k}} > c_{hk+1} > c_{hk}$ by the ordering of the initial treatment set and therefore $h\hat{k}$ cannot strongly dominate hk. And if the second pair of inequalities holds, $q_{hd} > q_{hk+1} > q_{h\hat{k}}$ also by the ordering of the initial treatment set, so that $h\hat{k}$ cannot strongly dominate treatment hd.

Proof of (ii): If $h\hat{k}$ does not strongly dominate hk-1, either $c_{h\hat{k}} > c_{hk-1}$, $q_{h\hat{k}} > q_{hk-1}$ or $c_{h\hat{k}} < c_{hk-1}$, $q_{h\hat{k}} < q_{hk-1}$. The second of the two pairs of inequalities is impossible because $q_{h\hat{k}} < q_{hk-1} < q_{hk}$ and $h\hat{k}$ does not strongly dominate hk. If the first pair of inequalities holds, $c_{h\hat{k}} > c_{hk-1} > c_{hd}$, so that $h\hat{k}$ cannot strongly dominate hd.

Lemma 4. Assume a new treatment $h\hat{k}$ is added to the treatment set for h and that it is not dominated. Then if $h\hat{k}$ strongly dominates an initial treatment hk for illness h but does not strongly or weakly dominate

(i) treatment hk+1, it does not weakly dominate any treatment hd such that d > k+1.

(ii) treatment hk-1, it does not weakly dominate any treatment hd such that d < k+1.

Proof of (i): If $h\hat{k}$ strongly dominates hk but not hk+1, it must be that $c_{hd} > c_{hk+1} > c_{h\hat{k}} \geq c_{hk}$ and thus, by the ordering of the initial treatment set, that $q_{hd} > q_{hk+1} > q_{h\hat{k}} \geq q_{hk}$. Hence if $h\hat{k}$ and some initial treatment hp weakly dominate hd, it must be that $c_{hp} > c_{hd} > c_{h\hat{k}}$, $q_{hp} > q_{hd} > q_{h\hat{k}}$, and by Proposition 2(iii),

$$\frac{c_{hp} - c_{h\hat{k}}}{q_{hp} - q_{h\hat{k}}} > \frac{c_{hp} - c_{hd}}{q_{hp} - q_{hd}}.$$

But by Lemma 2,

$$\frac{c_{hp} - c_{hd}}{q_{hp} - q_{hd}} > \frac{c_{hp} - c_{hk+1}}{q_{hp} - q_{hk+1}}$$

so that by Proposition 2(iii) $h\hat{k}$ and hp weakly dominate hk+1. This result contradicts the premise that the initial treatment set for h has no dominated members and it follows that $h\hat{k}$ cannot weakly dominate hd.

Proof of (ii): If $h\hat{k}$ strongly dominates hk but not hk-1, it must be that $q_{h\hat{k}} \geq q_{hk} > q_{hk-1} > q_{hd}$. Thus $c_{hk} \geq c_{h\hat{k}} > c_{hk-1} > c_{hd}$, and if hd is weakly dominated by $h\hat{k}$ and hp, it must also be that $c_{h\hat{k}} > c_{hd} > c_{hp}$ and $q_{h\hat{k}} > q_{hd} > q_{hp}$. Then if $h\hat{k}$ and hp weakly dominate hd, by Proposition 2(ii),

$$\frac{c_{hd} - c_{hp}}{q_{hd} - q_{hp}} \geq \frac{c_{h\hat{k}} - c_{hp}}{q_{h\hat{k}} - q_{hp}}.$$

But by Lemma 2,

$$\frac{c_{hk-1} - c_{hp}}{q_{k-1} - q_{hp}} \geq \frac{c_{h\hat{k}} - c_{hp}}{q_{h\hat{k}} - q_{hp}}$$

and by Proposition 2(ii) the inequality now implies that $h\hat{k}$ and hp weakly dominate hk-1.   The result contradicts the premise that hk-1 is not dominated, and therefore $\hat{hk}$ cannot weakly dominate hd.

Lemma 5. Assume a new treatment $\hat{hk}$ is added to the treatment set for h and that it is not dominated. Then if $\hat{hk}$ and some other treatment hp weakly dominate an initial treatment hk for illness h but $\hat{hk}$ does not strongly or weakly dominate

(i) treatment hk+1, it does not strongly dominate any treatment hd such that d > k+1.

(ii) treatment hk-1, it does not strongly dominate any treatment hd such that d < k+1.

Proof of (i): If $\hat{hk}$ and some initial treatment hp weakly dominate hk, either $c_{h\hat{k}} > c_{hk}$, $q_{h\hat{k}} > q_{hk}$ or $c_{h\hat{k}} < c_{hk}$, $q_{h\hat{k}} < q_{hk}$. Suppose $c_{h\hat{k}} > c_{hk}$ and $q_{h\hat{k}} > q_{hk}$. Then $c_{hk} > c_{hp}$, $q_{hk} > q_{hp}$, and by Proposition 2(ii),

$$\frac{c_{hk} - c_{hp}}{q_{hk} - q_{hp}} \geq \frac{c_{h\hat{k}} - c_{hp}}{q_{h\hat{k}} - q_{hp}}.$$

But if that is true, by Lemma 2,

$$\frac{c_{hk+1} - c_{hp}}{q_{hk+1} - q_{hp}} > \frac{c_{hk} - c_{hp}}{q_{hk} - q_{hp}} \text{ and } \frac{c_{hk+1} - c_{hp}}{q_{hk+1} - q_{hp}} > \frac{c_{h\hat{k}} - c_{hp}}{q_{h\hat{k}} - q_{hp}}.$$

Thus $\hat{hk}$ and hp weakly dominate hk+1, and on account of this contradiction of premise it must be that $c_{h\hat{k}} < c_{hk}$, $q_{h\hat{k}} < q_{hk}$. Therefore, by the ordering of the initial treatment set $q_{h\hat{k}} < q_{hk} < q_{hk+1} < q_{hd}$ and $\hat{hk}$ cannot strongly dominate hd.

Proof of (ii): Again, if $\hat{hk}$ and hp weakly dominate hk, either $c_{h\hat{k}} > c_{hk}$, $q_{h\hat{k}} > q_{hk}$ or $c_{h\hat{k}} < c_{hk}$, $q_{h\hat{k}} < q_{hk}$. If the second set of inequalities holds, $c_{hk} < c_{hp}$ and $q_{hk} < q_{hp}$, and by Proposition 2(iii),

$$\frac{c_{hp} - c_{h\hat{k}}}{q_{hp} - q_{h\hat{k}}} \geq \frac{c_{hp} - c_{hk}}{q_{hp} - q_{hk}}.$$

But in that case

$$\frac{c_{hp} - c_{hk}}{q_{hp} - q_{hk}} > \frac{c_{hp} - c_{hk-1}}{q_{hp} - q_{hk-1}}$$

by Lemma 2, so that

$$\frac{c_{hp} - c_{h\hat{k}}}{q_{hp} - q_{h\hat{k}}} > \frac{c_{hp} - c_{hk-1}}{q_{hp} - q_{hk-1}}$$

and therefore $h\hat{k}$ and hp weakly dominate hk-1. This result is another contradiction of premise, and it follows that $c_{h\hat{k}} > c_{hk}$, $q_{h\hat{k}} > q_{hk}$. Accordingly, by the ordering of the initial treatment set $c_{h\hat{k}} > c_{hk} > c_{hk-1} > c_{hd}$, and $h\hat{k}$ cannot strongly dominate hd.

Lemma 6. Assume a new treatment $h\hat{k}$ is added to the treatment set for h and that it is not dominated. Then if $h\hat{k}$ and some other treatment weakly dominate an initial treatment hk for illness h but $h\hat{k}$ does not strongly or weakly dominate

(i) treatment hk+1, it does not weakly dominate any treatment hd such that d > k+1.

(ii) treatment hk-1, it does not weakly dominate any treatment hd such that d < k+1.

Proof of (i): By the argument of the proof of Lemma 7(i) $c_{h\hat{k}} < c_{hk}$, $q_{h\hat{k}} < q_{hk}$. Suppose $h\hat{k}$ and some other treatment hp weakly dominate hd. Then by Proposition 2(iii), $c_{hd} < c_{hp}$, $q_{hd} < q_{hp}$, and

$$\frac{c_{hp} - c_{h\hat{k}}}{q_{hp} - q_{h\hat{k}}} \geq \frac{c_{hp} - c_{hd}}{q_{hp} - q_{hd}}.$$

But because d > k+1,

$$\frac{c_{hp} - c_{hd}}{q_{hp} - q_{hd}} > \frac{c_{hp} - c_{hk+1}}{q_{hp} - q_{hk+1}}$$

by Lemma 2, and as a consequence $h\hat{k}$ and hp also weakly dominate hk+1. This contradiction of premise implies that there is no hp such that it and $h\hat{k}$ weakly dominate hd.

Proof of (ii): By the argument of the proof of Lemma 5(ii) $c_{h\hat{k}} > c_{hk}$, $q_{h\hat{k}} > q_{hk}$. Suppose $h\hat{k}$ and some other treatment hp weakly dominate hd. Now $c_{h\hat{k}} > c_{hk} > c_{hp}$, $q_{h\hat{k}} > q_{hk} > q_{hp}$, and by Proposition 2(ii),

$$\frac{c_{hd} - c_{hp}}{q_{hd} - q_{hp}} \geq \frac{c_{h\hat{k}} - c_{hp}}{q_{h\hat{k}} - q_{hp}}.$$

However, because k-1 > d, Lemma 2 gives

$$\frac{c_{hk-1} - c_{hp}}{q_{hk-1} - q_{hp}} > \frac{c_{hd} - c_{hp}}{q_{hd} - q_{hp}} \geq \frac{c_{h\hat{k}} - c_{hp}}{q_{h\hat{k}} - q_{hp}},$$

treatment hk-1. This result contradicts the premise that hk-1 is not weakly dominated, and also by Proposition 2(ii) it must then be true that $h\hat{k}$ and hp weakly dominate and therefore there is no hp such that it and $h\hat{k}$ weakly dominate hd.

Lemmas 3-6 show that if $h\hat{k}$ (i) dominates hk but not hk+1, it does not dominate any hd such that d > k+1; and (ii) if it dominates hk but not hk-1, it does not dominate any hd such that d < k-1. The results are summarized in

Proposition 10. Let $h\hat{k}$ be a new treatment for h that it is not dominated. If $h\hat{k}$ dominates one or more of the initial treatments for illness h, the dominated treatments are an ordered subset of the initial treatment set having the form {hk, hk+1,..., hk*} with k ≤ k*, and the treatments in the subset are numbered in the same way as they are in the initial treatment set for h.

There remains the question of where treatment $h\hat{k}$ is placed in the new treatment set after the treatments it dominates are deleted. The next proposition answers that question. Treatment $h\hat{k}$ replaces the subset of treatments it dominates in the ordered set of treatments for h.

Proposition 11. Let $h\hat{k}$ be a new treatment for h that it is not dominated. Suppose $h\hat{k}$ dominates one or more of the initial treatments hk, hk+1,...,hk*, where k* ≥ k. Assume that these dominated treatments are removed from the treatment set. Then the new ordered treatment set is

(i) {h1, h2,..., hk-1, $h\hat{k}$, hk*+1,..., hK} if k* < K, and

102

(ii) $\{h1, h2, ..., hk-1, h\hat{k}\}$ if $k^* = K$.

Proof: When all treatments dominated by $h\hat{k}$ are removed from the treatment set for h, the new set (containing $h\hat{k}$) is ordered so that treatment costs and health benefits both strictly increase in the treatment index. By Proposition 10 the ordered subset of dominated treatments is $\{hk, hk+1,..., hk^*\}$. Thus by the proofs of parts (ii) of Lemmas 3-6, $c_{h\hat{k}} > c_{hk-1}$ and $q_{h\hat{k}} \geq q_{hk}$ whether $h\hat{k}$ strongly or weakly dominates hk, and therefore $\hat{k} > k-1$. Assume that there is a treatment hk*+1. Then by parts (i) of Lemmas 3-6, $c_{h\hat{k}} < c_{hk^*+1}$, $q_{h\hat{k}} < q_{hk^*+1}$ whether $h\hat{k}$ strongly or weakly dominates hk*, and as a consequence $\hat{k} < k^*+1$. Then $k-1 < \hat{k} < k^*+1$. Thus the revised treatment set has the form (i) if hk*+1 exists, and otherwise it has the form (ii). Observe that h1 is always a member of the revised treatment set because it cannot be dominated.

Assume a new treatment $h\hat{k}$ is not dominated by any of the initial treatments for h. The GM decision rules for assessing the absolute cost-effectiveness of $h\hat{k}$ are presented in the next section. Although the rules are simple ones, proving them requires effort because of the different structures the treatment set for h can take before and after $h\hat{k}$ is entered into it. There are eight such structures. First of all, the treatment set differs depending on whether h = i or h ≠ i. *Illness i will be called the cutoff-point illness* inasmuch as the two treatments that define the cutoff point in Proposition 8 are ij and ij-1. Second, and depending on whether and how $h\hat{k}$ dominates any of the initial treatments, there are four different structures of the treatment set for the cutoff-point illness and each non-cutoff-point illness. The section ends with a list of the four types and their properties.

1. **$h\hat{k}$ does not dominate any of the initial treatments for h and $R_{h\hat{k}} > R_{hK}$.** The new ordered treatment set is for h $\{h1, h2,..., hK, h\hat{k}\}$.

The placement of $h\hat{k}$ follows from Proposition 5. The treatments in the new nondominated set are ordered so that treatment costs, treatment health benefits, and the ICE ratios measured on adjacent treatments in the set all strictly increase in the treatment index.

2. **$h\hat{k}$ does not dominate any of the initial treatments for h and $R_{h\hat{k}} < R_{hK}$.** The new ordered treatment set for h is {h1, h2,..., hk-1, $h\hat{k}$, $h\hat{k}$ +1,..., hK}.

Because the new treatment set has no dominated members the ordering of the new treatment set follows from Proposition 5. Notice also that the ICE ratio

$$R_{hk} = \frac{c_{hk} - c_{hk-1}}{q_{hk} - q_{hk-1}}$$

is deleted from the initial ordered set of all ICE ratios and replaced by two new ratios,

(27) $$R_{h\hat{k}} = \frac{c_{h\hat{k}} - c_{hk-1}}{q_{h\hat{k}} - q_{hk-1}} \quad \text{and} \quad R_{h\hat{k}+1} = \frac{c_{hk} - c_{h\hat{k}}}{q_{hk} - q_{h\hat{k}}},$$

and $R_{h\hat{k}} < R_{hk} < R_{h\hat{k}+1}$. These two inequalities follow from (27). Specifically,

$$(c_{h\hat{k}} - c_{hk-1})(q_{hk} - q_{hk-1} + q_{hk-1} - q_{h\hat{k}}) <$$
$$(c_{hk} - c_{hk-1} + c_{hk-1} - c_{h\hat{k}})(q_{h\hat{k}} - q_{hk-1})$$

gives $R_{h\hat{k}} < R_{hk}$, and

$$(c_{h\hat{k}} - c_{hk} + c_{hk} - c_{hk-1})(q_{hk} - q_{h\hat{k}}) <$$
$$(c_{hk} - c_{h\hat{k}})(q_{h\hat{k}} - q_{hk} + q_{hk} - q_{hk-1})$$

gives $R_{hk} < R_{h\hat{k}+1}$.

3. **$h\hat{k}$ dominates one or more of the initial treatments for h and $R_{h\hat{k}} < R_{hK}$.**

By Proposition 10 the ordered subset of dominated treatments is {hk, hk+1,..., hm,..., hk*}. These treatments are deleted from the initial set of all treatments for all illnesses and the ICE ratios R_{hk}, $R_{hk+1},\ldots,$ $R_{hm},\ldots,$ R_{hk^*+1} are removed from the ordered set of all ICE ratios. By Proposition 11 the new treatment set for h is {h1, h2,..., hk-1, $h\hat{k}$, $h\hat{k}+1$,..., hK}. Observe in addition that two new ICE ratios are added to the ordered set of all ICE ratios,

$$R_{h\hat{k}} = \frac{c_{h\hat{k}} - c_{hk-1}}{q_{h\hat{k}} - q_{hk-1}} \text{ and } R_{h\hat{k}+1} = \frac{c_{hk^*+1} - c_{h\hat{k}}}{q_{hk^*+1} - q_{h\hat{k}}},$$

and $R_{h\hat{k}} \leq R_{hm} \leq R_{h\hat{k}+1}$ for all hm in the set of dominated treatments. Proving these two inequalities is a straightforward but length lengthy procedure, and because the proof is of no intrinsic interest it is given in the appendix to the chapter.

4. $h\hat{k}$ dominates one or more of the initial treatments for h and $R_{h\hat{k}} \geq R_{hK}$. Specifically, $h\hat{k}$ dominates only hK, the new ordered treatment set for h is {h1, h2,..., hK-1, $h\hat{k}$ }, and $R_{h\hat{k}} = R_{hK}$.

The form of the new treatment set and the relation between $R_{h\hat{k}}$ R_{hK} can be explained in this way. Assume all of the dominated treatments have been removed from the treatment set. Then by Proposition 11 the new treatment set is either {h1, h2,..., hk-1, $h\hat{k}$, hk*+1,..., hK} if k* < K or {h1, h2,..., hk-1, $h\hat{k}$} if k* = K. But it cannot be of the first form because the new set contains no dominated treatments by premise, that implies $R_{h\hat{k}} <$ R_{hK} by Proposition 5, and this inequality contradicts premise. Therefore, the treatment set must be of the second form so that $h\hat{k}$ dominates hK. But $h\hat{k}$ cannot strongly strictly dominate hK because if it does, $c_{h\hat{k}} < c_{hK}$, $q_{h\hat{k}} > q_{hK}$, and by Lemma 2,

$$R_{hK} = \frac{c_{hK} - c_{hK-1}}{q_{hK} - q_{hK-1}} \geq \frac{c_{hK} - c_{hk-1}}{q_{hK} - q_{hk-1}} > \frac{c_{h\hat{k}} - c_{hk-1}}{q_{h\hat{k}} - q_{hk-1}} = R_{h\hat{k}}.$$

Accordingly, the contradiction of premise implies that $h\hat{k}$ and some other nondominated treatment hp must weakly dominate hK. Inasmuch as there is no initial hp more costly and more health benefit productive than hK, it must also be that $c_{h\hat{k}} > c_{hK} > c_{hp}$, $q_{h\hat{k}} > q_{hK} > q_{hp}$. Hence by Lemma 2 and Proposition 2(i)

$$\frac{c_{hK} - c_{hK-1}}{q_{hK} - q_{hK-1}} \geq \frac{c_{hK} - c_{hp}}{q_{hK} - q_{hp}} \geq \frac{c_{h\hat{k}} - c_{hK}}{q_{h\hat{k}} - q_{hK}}.$$

As a result,

$$(c_{hk} - c_{hk-1})(q_{h\hat{k}} - q_{hK-1} + q_{hK-1} - q_{hK}) \geq$$
$$(c_{h\hat{k}} - c_{hK-1} + c_{hK-1} - c_{hK})(q_{hk} - q_{hK-1})$$

and

$$R_{hK} = \frac{c_{hK} - c_{hK-1}}{q_{hK} - q_{hK-1}} \geq \frac{c_{h\hat{k}} - c_{hK-1}}{q_{h\hat{k}} - q_{hK-1}} = R_{h\hat{k}}.$$

Thus it must be that $R_{hK} = R_{h\hat{k}}$.

At this point and because the placement of budget intervals has a central role in the proofs of the single-treatment decision rules of the next two sections, it is convenient to re-introduce and add to the terminology and notation used in the proof of Proposition 9.   Define the budget intervals

$B_{ij} = (C^{t-1}, C^t]$ initially associated with R_{ij},

$B_{ij}' = (C^{t-1}, C^{t'}]$ associated with R_{ij} after $h\hat{k}$ enters the treatment set,

$B_{h\hat{k}} = (C^{s-1}, C^s]$ associated with $R_{h\hat{k}}$ after $h\hat{k}$ enters the treatment set and all dominated treatments have been removed from the treatment set for h,

$B_{h\hat{k}+1} = (C^{s'-1}, C^{s'}]$ associated with $R_{h\hat{k}+1}$ after $h\hat{k}$ enters the treatment set and all dominated treatments have been removed from the treatment set for h.

It will be said that a budget interval is positioned or enters the ordered set of all budget intervals on the left or right side of some other budget interval. This means, for example, that if $B_{h\hat{k}}$ enters the ordered set of all budget intervals on, or is positioned on, the left of B_{ij}, $C^s \leq C^{t-1}$. Similarly, if $B_{h\hat{k}+1}$ enters the ordered set of all budget intervals on, or is positioned on, the right of $B_{ij}^{'}$, it means that $C^{t'} \leq C^{s'-1}$. To shorten the proofs this notation will also be used:

$B_{ij}^{'} \text{ E } B_{h\hat{k}}$ means that $B_{h\hat{k}}$ is positioned on the right of $B_{ij}^{'}$ ($B_{ij}^{'}$ is positioned on the left of $B_{h\hat{k}}$), and

$B_{ij}^{'} = B_{ij}$ means that $B_{ij}^{'}$ and B_{ij} are the same interval.

Recall that the ordering of all ICE ratios imposes an ordering on the set of all budget intervals such that $\rho_{hk} < \rho_{gm}$ implies $B_{hk} \text{ E } B_{gm}$.

Because they are used in the proofs of the rules for absolute cost-effectiveness, notice also that the new treatment sets of Types 2 and 3 have two commonalities. The first is that in both of them the deleted ICE ratios are bounded by $R_{h\hat{k}}$ and $R_{h\hat{k}+1}$. That is, $R_{h\hat{k}} < R_{hk} < R_{h\hat{k}+1}$ when hk is deleted and the set is of Type 2, and $R_{h\hat{k}} \leq R_{hm} \leq R_{h\hat{k}+1}$ for all deleted R_{hm} if the set is of Type 3. Hence $B_{h\hat{k}} \text{ E } B_{hk} \text{ E } B_{h\hat{k}+1}$ if the new set is of Type 2, and $B_{h\hat{k}} \text{ E } B_{hm} \text{ E } B_{h\hat{k}+1}$ for all deleted B_{hm} if the new set if of Type 3. The second property that both treatment sets share is that the total length of the budget intervals $B_{h\hat{k}}$ and $B_{h\hat{k}+1}$ added to the ordered set of all budget intervals equals the total length of the budget intervals that are deleted. Recall that the length of any budget interval B_{hk} associated with the ICE ratio

$$R_{hk} = \frac{c_{hk} - c_{hk-1}}{q_{hk} - q_{hk-1}}$$

Is $(c_{hk} - c_{hk-1})N_h$, where N_h is the number of patients having illness h. If the new treatment set is of Type 2, the budget interval B_{hk} is associated with the deleted ICE ratio R_{hk}, and $\text{length}(B_{h\hat{k}}) + \text{length}(B_{h\hat{k}+1}) =$ $(c_{h\hat{k}} - c_{hk-1})N_h + (c_{hk} - c_{h\hat{k}})N_h = (c_{hk} - c_{hk-1})N_h = \text{length}(B_{hk})$. When the new treatment set is of Type 3 the initial budget intervals $B_{hk}, B_{hk+1}, \ldots, B_{hk^*+1}$ are deleted. Therefore, $\text{length}(B_{h\hat{k}}) + \text{length}(B_{h\hat{k}+1}) = [((c_{hk} - c_{hk-1}) + (c_{hk+1} - c_{hk}) + \ldots + (c_{hk^*+1} - c_{hk^*})]N_h = \text{length}(\text{all deleted budget intervals})$.

4.3 The Decision Rules for Absolute Cost-effectiveness When $h \neq i$

Proposition 12. Let $h\hat{k}$ be a new nondominated treatment for $h = i$ or $h \neq i$. Add it to the treatment set for h and remove all treatments, if any, that it dominates. Assume $R_{h\hat{k}} \neq R(C)$. If there is a treatment $h\hat{k}+1$, assume also that $R_{h\hat{k}+1} \neq R(C)$ and that $C \neq C^t$ for all C. Then $h\hat{k}$ is not absolutely cost-effective (not optimal) for h if

$$R_{h\hat{k}} \neq \max_{m} \{R_{hm} < R(C)\},$$

where each hm is in the new treatment set for h.

Proof: First of all, $R(C) = R_{ij}$, and by the premises

$$R_{h\hat{k}} < \max_{m} \{R_{hm} < R(C)\}$$

implies $R_{h\hat{k}} < R_{ij}$, and if there is an $h\hat{k}+1$,

$$R_{h\hat{k}} > \max_{m} \{R_{hm} < R(C)\}$$

implies $R_{h\hat{k}} > R_{ij}$.

Assume the new treatment set is of Type 1 or Type 4. For each type of new treatment set there is no $h\hat{k}+1$, and it therefore cannot happen that

$$R_{h\hat{k}} < \max_{m} \{R_{hm} < R(C)\}.$$

So suppose

$$R_{h\hat{k}} > \max_{m} \{R_{hm} < R(C)\}.$$

Then the new budget interval $B_{h\hat{k}}$ enters the ordered set of all budget intervals on the right of B_{ij}, and there are no other changes in the ordered set. Therefore, the endpoints of B_{ij} are unchanged, $B_{ij}' = B_{ij}$, C is in B_{ij}, and because $R_{h\hat{k}} > R_{ij}$, $h\hat{k}$ is not absolutely cost-effective by (19) and (20) of Proposition 8.

Assume next the new treatment set is of Type 2 or 3 and suppose

$$R_{h\hat{k}} > \max_{m} \{R_{hm} < R(C)\}.$$

108

Then $B_{h\hat{k}}$ and $B_{h\hat{k}+1}$ are added to the ordered set of all budget intervals on the right of B_{ij}, and since $R_{ij} < R_{h\hat{k}} \leq R_{hm}$ for every deleted R_{hm}, each deleted budget interval B_{hm} is initially positioned on the right of B_{ij} as well. Therefore, adding $h\hat{k}$ to the treatment set for h leaves the endpoints of B_{ij} unchanged, C is in B_{ij}, and because $R_{h\hat{k}} > R_{ij}$, $h\hat{k}$ is not absolutely cost-effective by (19) and (20) of Proposition 8. Finally, suppose

$$R_{h\hat{k}} < \max_{m} \{R_{hm} < R(C)\}.$$

Accordingly, $R_{h\hat{k}} < R_{h\hat{k}+1} < R_{ij}$, $B_{h\hat{k}}$ and $B_{h\hat{k}+1}$ are added to the ordered set of all budget intervals on the left of B_{ij}. Then inasmuch as $R_{hm} \leq R_{h\hat{k}+1} < R_{ij}$ for each R_{hm}, the deleted budget intervals B_{hm} are also initially positioned on the left of B_{ij}. Because the lengths of the added and deleted budget intervals are equal for new treatments sets of Types 2 and 3 and $R_{h\hat{k}} < R_{h\hat{k}+1} < R_{ij}$, $h\hat{k}$ is not absolutely cost-effective by (19) and (20) of Proposition 8. This result concludes the proof.

The next several proofs make use of the claims of Proposition 9, and for that reason it is restated here: let $(C^{s-1}, C^s]$ be the budget interval associated with $R_{h\hat{k}}$ and treatment $h\hat{k}$. If there is a treatment $h\hat{k}+1$, let $(C^{s'-1}, C^{s'}]$ be the budget interval associated with $R_{h\hat{k}+1}$ and treatment $h\hat{k}+1$. Then if there is

(i) a treatment $h\hat{k}+1$, $h\hat{k}$ is optimal for illness h at all C such that $C^{s-1} < C < C^{s'}$.

(ii) no treatment $h\hat{k}+1$, $h\hat{k}$ is optimal for illness h at all $C > C^{s-1}$.

Proposition 13. Let $h\hat{k}$ be a new nondominated treatment for h. Add $h\hat{k}$ to the treatment set for h and remove all treatments, if any, that it dominates. Assume that $R_{h\hat{k}} \neq R(C)$. If there is a treatment $h\hat{k}+1$, assume also that $R_{h\hat{k}+1} \neq R(C)$ and that $C \neq C^t$ for all C. Then $h\hat{k}$ is absolutely cost-effective (optimal) for h if and only if

(28) $$R_{h\hat{k}} = \max_{m} \{R_{hm} < R(C)\},$$

where each hm is in the new treatment set for h.

Proof: Necessity of the proposition's claim is given by Proposition 12, and the proof establishes sufficiency of the claim. So assume

$$R_{h\hat{k}} = \max_{m} \{R_{hm} < R(C)\}$$

and suppose the new ordered treatment set is of Type 1 or Type 4: i.e., it is $\{h1, h2,..., h\hat{k}-1, h\hat{k}\}$, where $h\hat{k}-1 = hK$ if the set is of Type 1 and $h\hat{k}-1 = hK-1$ if it is of Type 4. Then since $R_{h\hat{k}} < R(C) = R_{ij}$, $B_{h\hat{k}}$ enters the ordered set of all budget intervals on the left of B_{ij} and displaces the endpoints of B_{ij} rightward to those of B_{ij}' by length($B_{h\hat{k}}$) = $C^s - C^{s-1}$. That is, $C'^{t-1} = C^{t-1} + C^s - C^{s-1}$, and $C^{t'} = C^t + C^s - C^{s-1}$. Next, $R_{h\hat{k}} < R_{ij}$ implies $B_{h\hat{k}} \mathrm{E} B_{ij}'$ so that $C^s \le C'^{t-1}$ (the relation is an inequality because there may be intervals positioned between $B_{h\hat{k}}$ and B_{ij}'), and

$$C^s \le C'^{t-1} = C^{t-1} + \text{length}(B_{h\hat{k}}) < C + C^s - C^{s-1}.$$

Thus $C^{s-1} < C$ and $h\hat{k}$ is therefore absolutely cost-effective by Proposition 9(ii).

If the new treatment set is of either Type 2 or Type 3, the new ordered treatment set is $\{h1, h2,..., hk-1, h\hat{k}, h\hat{k}+1,..., hK\}$, where hk is deleted from the initial ordered set when the new set is of Type 2 and the dominated treatments $hk, hk+1,..., hk*$ are deleted when the new set is of Type 3. In addition, $R_{h\hat{k}} < R_{hk} < R_{h\hat{k}+1}$ if the new treatment set is of Type 2, and $R_{h\hat{k}} \le R_{hk} < R_{hk+1} < \cdots < R_{hk*} \le R_{h\hat{k}+1}$ for the dominated and deleted treatments $hk, hk+1,..., hk*$ if it is of Type 3. Again assume

$$R_{h\hat{k}} = \max_{m} \{R_{hm} < R(C)\}.$$

Hence $R(C) = R_{ij}$ and by premise $R_{h\hat{k}} < R_{ij} < R_{h\hat{k}+1}$. If the new treatment set is of Type 2, R_{hk} is removed from the ordered set of all ICE ratios and B_{hk} is removed from the ordered set of all budget intervals. $R_{h\hat{k}} < R_{hk} < R_{h\hat{k}+1}$ implies $B_{h\hat{k}} \mathrm{E} B_{hk} \mathrm{E} B_{h\hat{k}+1}$ before B_{hk} is deleted, and length(B_{hk}) = length($B_{h\hat{k}}$) + length($B_{h\hat{k}+1}$). Adding $h\hat{k}$ to the treatment set for h consequently causes the left endpoint C^{t-1} of B_{ij} to be displaced to C'^{t-1} by

110

at most length($B_{h\hat{k}}$) = $C^s - C^{s-1}$ (at most this distance because B_{hk} or other intervals may be positioned between $B_{h\hat{k}}$ and B_{ij}). Since $B_{h\hat{k}}$ E B_{ij}', $C^s \le$ C^{t-1}, and these inequalities give $C^s \le C^{t-1} \le C^t + C^s - C^{s-1}$ whence $C^{s-1} <$ C. Next, the right endpoint C^t of B_{ij} is displaced to $C^{t'}$ by at least length($B_{h\hat{k}}$) − length(B_{hk}) = - length($B_{h\hat{k}+1}$) = $C^{s-1} - C^{s'}$ (at least this distance because B_{hk} may be positioned on the left of B_{ij}). B_{ij}' E $B_{h\hat{k}+1}$ implies $C^{t'} \le C^{s-1}$, so that $C^{s-1} \ge C^{t'} \ge C^t + C^{s-1} - C^s$, and $C^s \ge C^t > C$. Altogether then, this reasoning shows that $C^{s-1} < C < C^{s'}$, and $h\hat{k}$ is therefore absolutely cost-effective by Proposition 9(i).

   With very minor qualifications the same argument applies if the new treatment set is of Type 3. Depending on how $R_{h\hat{k}}$, R_{hk} and R_{hk^*}, $R_{h\hat{k}+1}$ are ranked in the prioritization procedure it can happen that B_{hk} E $B_{h\hat{k}}$ or $B_{h\hat{k}+1}$ E B_{hk^*+1} but not both. Even so, it is still true that adding $h\hat{k}$ to the treatment set for h and removing the dominated members of the set displaces the left endpoint C^{t-1} of B_{ij} to $C^{t'-1}$ by at most length($B_{h\hat{k}}$) and the right endpoint C^t to $C^{t'}$ by at least length($B_{h\hat{k}}$) − length(all deleted budget intervals) = - length($B_{h\hat{k}+1}$). Thus $C^{s-1} < C < C^{s'}$ if $C < C^t$, and $h\hat{k}$ is absolutely cost-effective by Proposition 9(i). This result completes the proof.

Proposition 14. Let $h\hat{k}$ be a new nondominated treatment for h. Add it to the treatment set for h and remove all treatments, if any, that it dominates. Assume that $C \ne C^t$ for all C. Then if $R_{h\hat{k}}$ = R(C), $h\hat{k}$ can be declared absolutely cost-effective or not as the health care agency prefers, and each option yields the same optimal total quantity of health benefits.

Proof: Since $R_{h\hat{k}}$ = R(C) = R_{ij}, $R_{h\hat{k}}$ and R_{ij} can ranked in any way in the ordered set of all budget intervals, and by Corollary 8 the order in which they are ranked does change the optimal total quantity of health benefits. The proof here shows that $h\hat{k}$ can be made absolutely cost-effective or not by arbitrarily changing the order of the ranks. It follows that the health care agency or other user of the CEA can declare $h\hat{k}$ absolutely cost-effective or not as it prefers and with no loss of total health benefits. The proof of the proposition is largely similar to the proof of Proposition 13 and for that reason it is only sketched.

If the new treatment set is of Type 1 and $\rho_{ij} < \rho_{h\hat{k}}$, adding $h\hat{k}$ to the treatment set for h causes only the addition of $B_{h\hat{k}}$ to the ordered set of all budget intervals, and $B_{ij} \in B_{h\hat{k}}$. The endpoints of B_{ij} are unchanged, C is in B_{ij}, and $h\hat{k}$ is not absolutely cost-effective by (19) and (20) of Proposition 8. If $\rho_{ij} > \rho_{h\hat{k}}$, $B_{h\hat{k}} \in B_{ij}$, and $C^{s-1} = C^{t-1}$. Inasmuch as there is no $h\hat{k} + 1$, $h\hat{k}$ is absolutely cost-effective by Proposition 9(ii).

The proofs of the proposition for Types 2 and 3 new treatment sets are similar. If the new treatment set is of Type 2 and $\rho_{ij} < \rho_{h\hat{k}}$, $R_{h\hat{k}} < R_{hk} < R_{h\hat{k}+1}$ so that $B_{ij} \in B_{h\hat{k}} \in B_{hk} \in B_{h\hat{k}+1}$. Once more, adding $h\hat{k}$ to the treatment set for h does not change the endpoints of B_{ij} and $h\hat{k}$ is not absolutely cost-effective by (19) and (20) of Proposition 8. If the new treatment set is of Type 3, $R_{h\hat{k}} \leq R_{hk}$ but if $R_{h\hat{k}} = R_{hk}$ the rankings of R_{ij}, $R_{h\hat{k}}$, and R_{hk} can be set arbitrarily as $\rho_{ij} < \rho_{h\hat{k}} < \rho_{hk}$ or $\rho_{ij} < \rho_{hk} < \rho_{h\hat{k}}$ without changing the total quantity of health benefits. In each case the added budget intervals $B_{h\hat{k}}$, $B_{h\hat{k}+1}$, and all of the deleted intervals B_{hk}, $B_{hk+1}, \ldots$, B_{hk^*+1} are or can be positioned on the right of B_{ij} without changing the total quantity of health benefits. The endpoints of B_{ij} are then unchanged and $h\hat{k}$ is not absolutely cost-effective by (19) and (20) of Proposition 8. If $\rho_{ij} > \rho_{h\hat{k}}$, adding $h\hat{k}$ to the treatment set displaces C^{t-1} to C^{t-1} by at most length($B_{h\hat{k}}$) and C^t to $C^{t'}$ by at least length(deleted interval(s)) whether the set is of Type 2 or Type 3. Hence by the reasoning of the proof of Proposition 13, $C^{s-1} < C < C^{s'}$ and if $C < C^t$, $h\hat{k}$ is absolutely cost-effective for h by Proposition 9(i).

Finally, if the new treatment set is of Type 4, $h\hat{k}$ dominates only hK and $R_{h\hat{k}} = R_{hK} = R_{ij}$. If $\rho_{ij} < \rho_{h\hat{k}}$, $B_{h\hat{k}}$ and B_{hK} can therefore both be placed on the right of B_{ij}. Adding $h\hat{k}$ to the treatment set for h leaves the endpoints of B_{ij} unchanged, and $h\hat{k}$ is not absolutely cost-effective by (9) and (20) of Proposition 8. If $\rho_{ij} > \rho_{h\hat{k}}$, $B_{h\hat{k}}$ and B_{hK} can both be placed on the left of B_{ij}, and as a consequence the left endpoint of B_{ij} is displaced from C^{t-1} to C'^{t-1} by at most length($B_{h\hat{k}}$). By the previously given argument, $C^{s-1} < C$, and if $C < C^t$, $h\hat{k}$ is absolutely cost-effective for h by Proposition 9(ii).

Proposition 15. Let $h\hat{k}$ be a new nondominated treatment for h. Add it to the treatment set for h and remove all treatments, if any, that it dominates. Assume that $C \neq C^t$ for all C. Then if $R_{h\hat{k}+1} = R(C)$, $h\hat{k}$ can be declared absolutely cost-effective or not as the health care agency prefers, and each option yields the same optimal total quantity of health benefits.

Proof: The proof is closely similar to the proof of Proposition 14 except that the interchanged ranks are those of $R_{h\hat{k}+1}$ and, since there exists a treatment $h\hat{k}+1$, R_{hk*+1}. Thus the new treatment set must be of Types 2 or 3. The total optimal quantity of health benefits is the same by Corollary 8 regardless of the rank order of $R_{h\hat{k}+1}$ and R_{ij}, and it only needs to be shown that $h\hat{k}$ is or is not absolutely cost-effective depending on the arbitrary ranking of $R_{h\hat{k}+1}$ and R_{ij}.

Suppose $\rho_{ij} < \rho_{h\hat{k}+1}$. Then since $R_{h\hat{k}} < R_{h\hat{k}+1} = R(C) = R_{ij}$, $\rho_{h\hat{k}} < \rho_{ij} < \rho_{h\hat{k}+1}$. Hence $B_{h\hat{k}}$ E B_{ij} E $B_{h\hat{k}+1}$ for each of the two types of new treatment sets. Adding $h\hat{k}$ to the treatment set for h displaces the endpoints of B_{ij} to those of B'_{ij} by at most length($B_{h\hat{k}}$) and at least by – length(deleted budget interval(s)). Therefore, as in the proofs of Propositions 12 and 13, $C^{s-1} < C < C^{s'}$ if $C < C^t$, and $h\hat{k}$ is absolutely cost-effective for h by Proposition 9(i). Next suppose $\rho_{ij} > \rho_{h\hat{k}+1}$. Then $B_{h\hat{k}}$ E $B_{h\hat{k}+1}$ E B_{ij}. When the new treatment set is of Type 2, $R_{h\hat{k}} < R_{hk} < R_{h\hat{k}+1}$ so that the single deleted budget interval B_{hk} is also positioned on the left of B_{ij}. Because length(B_{hk}) = length($B_{h\hat{k}}$) + length($B_{h\hat{k}+1}$), it follows that $B'_{ij} = B_{ij}$. Total cost C is in B_{ij}, and because

$$p_{h\hat{k}+1} = \max_m \{p_{hm} < p_{ij}\},$$

$h\hat{k}+1$ is absolutely cost-effective for h by (19) and (20) of Proposition 8 and $h\hat{k}$ is not.

When the new treatment set is of Type 3, $R_{hk^*+1} \leq R_{h\hat{k}+1}$, and if $R_{hk^*+1} < R_{h\hat{k}+1}$ all of the deleted ICE ratios are smaller than $R_{h\hat{k}+1}$ and all of the deleted budget intervals $B_{hk}, B_{hk+1}, \ldots, B_{hk^*+1}$ are initially positioned on the left of B_{ij}. Hence once more $B'_{ij} = B_{ij}$ and $h\hat{k}$ is not absolutely cost-effective by (19) and (20) of Proposition 8. Moreover, the result is the same even if $R_{hk^*+1} = R_{h\hat{k}+1}$ because the two ratios can be ranked so that $p_{hk^*+1} < p_{h\hat{k}+1}$ without changing the optimal total quantity of health benefits. Thus it is still true that $B_{h\hat{k}}$, $B_{h\hat{k}+1}$, and all the deleted budget intervals are or can be positioned on the left of B_{ij}, and as a consequence it is still true that $h\hat{k}$ is not absolutely cost-effective by (19) and (20) of Proposition 8. The proof is now complete.

4.4 The Decision Rules for Absolute Cost-effectiveness When h = i

The analyst may or may not know whether or not the focal illness is the cutoff-point illness, but that knowledge is not necessary for deciding the absolute cost-effectiveness of $i\hat{k}$. In this section it is shown that the maximum ICE-ratio rule given in Proposition 13 is applicable whether or not the focal illness is also the health care system's cutoff-point illness. There are, however, no counterparts of Propositions 14 and 15. This is because—as in the previous section—all dominated treatments are assumed to be removed from the new treatment set before the ICE-ratio rules are applied. Lemmas 7 and 8 given below state that if

$$R_{i\hat{k}} = \frac{c_{i\hat{k}} - c_{i\hat{k}-1}}{q_{i\hat{k}} - q_{i\hat{k}-1}} = \frac{c_{ij} - c_{ij-1}}{q_{ij} - q_{ij-1}} \text{ or } R_{i\hat{k}+1} = \frac{c_{i\hat{k}+1} - c_{i\hat{k}}}{q_{i\hat{k}+1} - q_{i\hat{k}}} = \frac{c_{ij} - c_{ij-1}}{q_{ij} - q_{ij-1}},$$

one of the treatments on which the ICE ratios are defined is nonstrictly dominated. Thus the dominated treatment is first removed from the new treatment set and it cannot happen that $R_{i\hat{k}} = R(C)$ or $R_{i\hat{k}+1} = R(C)$. Since the removal is made during the first part of the CEA, it is unnecessary for analyst to know or be aware that the $R_{h\hat{k}} = R(C)$ and $R_{h\hat{k}+1} = R(C)$ decision rules are inapplicable when $h = i$.

Proposition 16. Let $i\hat{k}$ be a new nondominated treatment for illness i. Add it to the treatment set for i and remove all treatments, if any, that it dominates. Assume that $R_{i\hat{k}} \neq R(C)$. If there is a treatment $i\hat{k} + 1$, assume also that $R_{i\hat{k}+1} \neq R(C)$ and that $C < C^t$. Then $i\hat{k}$ is absolutely cost-effective (optimal) for i if and only if

(29) $R_{i\hat{k}} = \max_m \{R_{im} < R(C)\}$,

where each im is in the new treatment set for i.

Proof: Necessity of the premises is established by Proposition 12, so here it only needs to be shown that the premises are also sufficient. First of all, $R(C) = R_{ij}$ and if

$$R_{i\hat{k}} = \max_m \{R_{im} < R(C)\} \text{ and } R_{i\hat{k}}, R_{i\hat{k}+1} \neq R(C),$$

then $R_{i\hat{k}} < R_{ij} < R_{i\hat{k}+1}$. Notice that the premises preclude the possibility that the new treatment set is of Types 1 or 4. This is so because $R_{i\hat{k}} \geq R_{iK} \geq R_{ij}$ for each of the two types of treatment sets.

Suppose the new treatment set is of Type 2. That is, the set is $\{i1, i2, \ldots, ik-1, i\hat{k}, i\hat{k} +1, \ldots, iK\}$,

$$R_{i\hat{k}} = \frac{C_{i\hat{k}} - C_{ik}}{q_{i\hat{k}} - q_{ik}} < R_{ik} = \frac{C_{ik} - C_{ik-1}}{q_{ik} - q_{ik-1}} < \frac{C_{ik} - C_{i\hat{k}}}{q_{ik} - q_{i\hat{k}}} = R_{i\hat{k}+1},$$

and length($B_{i\hat{k}}$) + length($B_{i\hat{k}+1}$) = length(B_{ik}). Since R_{ij} is the only ICE ratio bounded from below and above by $R_{i\hat{k}}$ and $R_{i\hat{k}+1}$, and $R_{i\hat{k}} < R_{ij} < R_{i\hat{k}+1}$, it must be that ik = ij. Thus B_{ij} is the only budget interval to be deleted from the ordered set of all budget intervals. However, let $B_{i\hat{k}}$ be added to the ordered set of all budget interval before B_{ij} is removed. Then the endpoints of B_{ij} are displaced to those of B'_{ij} by length($B_{i\hat{k}}$) = $C^s - C^{s-1}$, and as in the proofs of Propositions 13-15 it follows that $C^{s-1} < C$. Now delete B_{ij} and add $B_{i\hat{k}+1}$ to the ordered set of all budget intervals. Accordingly, $C^{s-1} \geq C^{t-1}$ and $C^{s} = C^{s-1} + \text{length}(B_{i\hat{k}+1})$ so that

$$C^{s} \geq C^{t-1} + \text{length}(B_{i\hat{k}+1}) = C^{t-1} + \text{length}(B_{i\hat{k}}) +$$
$$\text{length}(B_{i\hat{k}+1}) = C^{t-1} + C^{t} - C^{t-1} = C^{t} > C.$$

Therefore, $C^{s-1} < C < C^{s}$ and $i\hat{k}$ is absolutely cost-effective by Proposition 9(i).

Next suppose the new treatment set is of Type 3. Then the initial treatments ik, ik+1,..., ik* are dominated and $R_{i\hat{k}} \leq R_{im} \leq R_{i\hat{k}+1}$ for all m = k, k+1,..., k*+1. It may be that $R_{i\hat{k}} = R_{ik}$ or $R_{i\hat{k}+1} = R_{ik*+1}$, but on account of the ordering of the initial set of ICE ratios defined on treatments for i there are no other equalities. The only ICE ratios bounded from below and above by $R_{i\hat{k}}$ and $R_{i\hat{k}+1}$ are those defined on the im, and as a result it must be that ij is a dominated treatment.

Add $B_{i\hat{k}}$ to the ordered set of all budget intervals and delete all the budget intervals B_{ik}, B_{ik+1},..., B_{ik*+1} except B_{ij}. As in the proofs of Propositions 13-15, the endpoints of B_{ij} are displaced to those of B_{ij}' by at most $\text{length}(B_{i\hat{k}})$, and again it can be concluded that $C^{s-1} < C$. Now add $B_{i\hat{k}+1}$ to the ordered set of all budget intervals and let $B_{i\hat{k}+1} = (C^{s-1}, C^{s}]$ before B_{ij} is removed from it. That is, $C^{s-1} = C^{s-1} - \text{length}(B_{ij})$ and $C^{s} = C^{s} - \text{length}(B_{ij})$. Thus as in the proofs of Propositions 13-15, $B_{ij}' E B_{i\hat{k}+1}$ because $R_{ij} < R_{i\hat{k}+1}$ so that

$$C^{s-1} \geq C^{t} - \text{length (all deleted intervals except } B_{ij}) =$$
$$C^{t} - \text{length (all deleted intervals)} + \text{length}(B_{ij}),$$

where the inequality occurs because it can happen that $R_{ik*+1} = R_{i\hat{k}+1}$ and $B_{ik*+1} E B_{i\hat{k}+1}$. Accordingly,

$$C^{s} = C^{s-1} + \text{length}(B_{i\hat{k}+1}) \geq [C^{t} + \text{length}(B_{i\hat{k}})] - [\text{length}(B_{i\hat{k}}) +$$
$$\text{length}(B_{i\hat{k}+1})] + \text{length}(B_{ij}) = C^{t} + \text{length}(B_{ij}),$$

and therefore $C^{s'} = C^{s''}$ - length(B_{ij}) $\geq C^t > C$. The argument has now shown that $C^{s-1} < C < C^{s'}$, and as a consequence $i\hat{k}$ is absolutely cost-effective by Proposition 9(i). This result completes the proof.

As said at the beginning of the section, there are no $R_{h\hat{k}} = R(C)$ or $R_{h\hat{k}+1} = R(C)$ decision rules when h = i because neither equality can occur. The section closes with a pair of lemmas showing that each of the two equalities implies that one of the treatments on which $R_{i\hat{k}}$, $R_{i\hat{k}1}$, and $R_{ij} = R(C)$ are defined is always weakly dominated. Thus when all dominated treatments are first removed from the new treatment set, it cannot happen that $R_{h\hat{k}} = R(C)$ or $R_{h\hat{k}+1} = R(C)$

Lemma 7. If $R_{i\hat{k}} = R(C)$, $i\hat{k}$ is dominated or it and ij-1 nonstrictly weakly dominate ij.

Proof: Add $i\hat{k}$ to the treatment set for i and remove all members of the treatment set that it strictly dominates. Order the remaining members of the set so that treatment costs and health benefits increase strictly in the treatment index. Assume

$$R_{i\hat{k}} = \frac{c_{i\hat{k}} - c_{i\hat{k}-1}}{q_{i\hat{k}} - q_{i\hat{k}-1}} = \frac{c_{ij} - c_{ij-1}}{q_{ij} - q_{ij-1}} = R(C).$$

Because $i\hat{k}$ -1 is by premise the costliest, most health-benefit productive treatment next to $i\hat{k}$, there are only four possible orderings of the new treatment set:

(i) $\{i1, i2,..., i\hat{k}$ -1, $i\hat{k}$,..., ij-1, ij,..., iK$\}$,

(ii) $(i1, i2,..., i\hat{k}$ -1, $i\hat{k}$, ij,..., iK$\}$ and $i\hat{k}$ -1 = ij-1,

(iii) $\{i1, i2,..., ij, i\hat{k}$,..., iK$\}$ and $i\hat{k}$ -1 = ij,

(iv) $\{i1, i2,..., ij,..., i\hat{k}$ -1, $i\hat{k}$,..., iK$\}$.

If the new treatment set has the ordering (i), by Lemma 2 applied to the initial treatment set,

$$\frac{c_{i\hat{k}} - c_{i\hat{k}-1}}{q_{i\hat{k}} - q_{i\hat{k}-1}} = \frac{c_{ij} - c_{ij-1}}{q_{ij} - q_{ij-1}} > \frac{c_{ij} - c_{i\hat{k}-1}}{q_{ij} - q_{i\hat{k}-1}}.$$

Hence by Proposition 2(ii) the inequality between then leftmost and rightmost ratios implies that ij and $i\hat{k}$ -1 strictly weakly dominate $i\hat{k}$. If (ii) is the ordering,

$$\frac{c_{i\hat{k}} - c_{ij-1}}{q_{i\hat{k}} - q_{ij-1}} = \frac{c_{ij} - c_{ij-1}}{q_{ij} - q_{ij-1}},$$

and by Proposition 2(ii) ij and ij-1 = $i\hat{k}$ -1 nonstrictly weakly dominate $i\hat{k}$. If (iii) is the ordering,

$$\frac{c_{i\hat{k}} - c_{ij}}{q_{i\hat{k}} - q_{ij}} = \frac{c_{ij} - c_{ij-1}}{q_{ij} - q_{ij-1}}$$

and by Proposition 2(i) $i\hat{k}$ and ij-1 nonstrictly weakly dominate ij.

Finally, suppose the treatment ordering is (iv). By Lemma 2 applied to the initial treatment set,

$$\frac{c_{i\hat{k}} - c_{i\hat{k}-1}}{q_{i\hat{k}} - q_{i\hat{k}-1}} = \frac{c_{ij} - c_{ij-1}}{q_{ij} - q_{ij-1}} < \frac{c_{i\hat{k}-1} - c_{ij-1}}{q_{i\hat{k}-1} - q_{ij-1}}$$

By Proposition 2(i) the inequality between the leftmost and rightmost ratios implies that $i\hat{k}$ and ij strictly weakly dominate $i\hat{k}$ -1. Hence $i\hat{k}$ -1 will be removed from the new treatment set before any operations are performed on the set, and as a result the ordering (iv) cannot occur. Therefore, the only possible orderings of the new treatment set are (i)-(iii), and in each of them $i\hat{k}$ is either weakly dominated or else it and ij-1 nonstrictly weakly dominate ij. The proof is now complete.

Lemma 8. If $R_{i\hat{k}+1}$ = R(C), $i\hat{k}$ is dominated or else it and ij nonstrictly weakly dominate treatment ij-1.

Proof: Let $i\hat{k}$ be added to the treatment set for illness i and assume that all treatments strictly dominated by $i\hat{k}$ are removed from the set. Assume the set has been ordered so that treatment costs and health benefits increase strictly in the treatment index and that the ICE ratios defined on adjacent treatments in the ordered set are nondecreasing in the treatment index. Assume that

$$R_{i\hat{k}+1} = \frac{c_{i\hat{k}+1} - c_{i\hat{k}}}{q_{i\hat{k}+1} - q_{i\hat{k}}} = R(C) = \frac{c_{ij} - c_{ij-1}}{q_{ij} - q_{ij-1}}.$$

118

Because $i\hat{k}$ is by premise the costliest, most health-benefit productive treatment next to $i\hat{k}+1$, there are only four possible orderings of the new treatment set:

(i) $\{i1, i2,\ldots, i\hat{k}, i\hat{k}+1,\ldots, ij\text{-}1, ij,\ldots, iK\}$,

(ii) $\{i1, i2,\ldots, i\hat{k}, i\hat{k}+1, ij,\ldots, iK\}$ and $i\hat{k}+1 = ij\text{-}1$,

(iii) $\{i1, i2,\ldots, i\hat{k}, i\hat{k}+1,\ldots, iK\}$ and $i\hat{k}+1 = ij$,

(iv) $\{i1, i2,\ldots, ij, \ldots, i\hat{k}, i\hat{k}+1,\ldots, iK\}$.

Suppose (i) is the ordered treatment set. Applying Lemma 2 to the initial treatment set with $ij\text{-}1 > i\hat{k}$ and then exploiting the ordering of ICE ratios defined on treatments in the new treatment set gives

$$\frac{c_{i\hat{k}+1} - c_{i\hat{k}}}{q_{i\hat{k}+1} - q_{i\hat{k}}} = \frac{c_{ij} - c_{ij\text{-}1}}{q_{ij} - q_{ij\text{-}1}} > \frac{c_{ij\text{-}1} - c_{i\hat{k}+1}}{q_{ij\text{-}1} - q_{ik+1}} \geq \frac{c_{i\hat{k}+1} - c_{i\hat{k}}}{q_{i\hat{k}+1} - q_{i\hat{k}}}.$$

The inequality between the leftmost and rightmost ratios gives a contradiction, and the ordered treatment set (i) therefore cannot occur.

If the new treatment set has the ordering (ii),

$$\frac{c_{i\hat{k}+1} - c_{i\hat{k}}}{q_{i\hat{k}+1} - q_{i\hat{k}}} = \frac{c_{ij\text{-}1} - c_{i\hat{k}}}{q_{ij\text{-}1} - q_{i\hat{k}}} = \frac{c_{ij} - c_{ij\text{-}1}}{q_{ij} - q_{ij\text{-}1}},$$

and by Proposition 2(i) $i\hat{k}$ and ij nonstrictly weakly dominate $ij\text{-}1 = i\hat{k}+1$. If the new treatment set has the ordering (iii),

$$\frac{c_{i\hat{k}+1} - c_{i\hat{k}}}{q_{i\hat{k}+1} - q_{i\hat{k}}} = \frac{c_{ij} - c_{i\hat{k}}}{q_{ij} - q_{i\hat{k}}} = \frac{c_{ij} - c_{ij\text{-}1}}{q_{ij} - q_{ij\text{-}1}},$$

and by Proposition 2(i) $ij = i\hat{k}+1$ and $ij\text{-}1$ nonstrictly weakly dominate $i\hat{k}$. Last of all, if the new treatment set has the ordering (iv), Lemma 2 applied to the new treatment set gives

$$\frac{c_{ij} - c_{ij\text{-}1}}{q_{ij} - q_{ij\text{-}1}} = \frac{c_{i\hat{k}+1} - c_{i\hat{k}}}{q_{i\hat{k}+1} - q_{i\hat{k}}} \geq \frac{c_{i\hat{k}} - c_{i\hat{k}\text{-}1}}{q_{i\hat{k}} - c_{i\hat{k}\text{-}1}} \geq \frac{c_{ij} - c_{ij\text{-}1}}{q_{ij} - q_{ij\text{-}1}}.$$

Hence

$$\frac{c_{i\hat{k}+1} - c_{i\hat{k}}}{q_{i\hat{k}+1} - q_{i\hat{k}}} = \frac{c_{i\hat{k}} - c_{i\hat{k}\text{-}1}}{q_{i\hat{k}} - c_{i\hat{k}\text{-}1}}$$

and by Proposition 2(i) the initial treatments $i\hat{k}+1$ and $i\hat{k}-1$ nonstrictly weakly dominate $i\hat{k}$.

In sum, the only possible orderings of the new treatment set are (ii)-

(iv), and for these orderings $i\hat{k}$ is either weakly dominated or it nonstrictly weakly dominates ij-1. The proof is now complete.

4.5 Summary of the Global Maximizer's Single-Treatment Decision Rules

To make the single-treatment decision rules obtained in Propositions 12-16 easier to refer to in the remaining chapters of the book, they are summarized here in Proposition 17. The rules are applicable to all four types of new treatment sets and to both cutoff-point and non-cutoff-point illnesses.

Proposition 17. Let $h\hat{k}$ be a new nondominated treatment for h, where h may or may not be the cutoff-point illness i. Let $R(C) = R_{ij}$, and assume $C \neq C^t$. Add $h\hat{k}$ to the treatment set for h and remove all treatments that it dominates. Then provided $C \neq C^t$ and

(i) $R_{h\hat{k}} = R(C)$, or if there is a treatment $h\hat{k} +1$, $R_{h\hat{k}+1} = R(C)$, $h\hat{k}$ can be declared absolutely cost-effective or not as the health care agency prefers, and each option yields the same total optimal quantity of health benefits.

(ii) $R_{h\hat{k}} \neq R(C)$, or if there is a treatment $h\hat{k} +1$ and $R_{h\hat{k}+1} \neq R(C)$, $h\hat{k}$ is absolutely cost-effective for illness h if and only if

(28) $$R_{h\hat{k}} = \max_{m} \{R_{hm} < R(C)\}.$$

There remains the qualification in Proposition 17 that the GM decision rules are not necessarily valid if $C = C^t$, and an example is given in Chapter 6 in which the rules do give an incorrect conclusion. Conditions exist that make the rules valid even if $C = C^t$, but they are of little or no use to analysts because they are not usually observable in practice. The $C \neq C^t$ qualification in Proposition 17 is therefore a theoretical limitation of single-treatment GM CEA, but the event that $C = C^t$ is so unlikely that as a practical matter it can be ignored.

To see this, consider that an analyst will almost certainly not know the health care agency's budget points even if he knows the agency's total treatment cost. Hence from the analyst's perspective the event that C equals any budget point can be taken as random. Treatment cost can be thought of as a random variable, and a CEA's conclusion can be regarded as possibly incorrect only if total treatment cost C equals the budget point C^t. Thus assessing the likelihood that the conclusion is wrong can be cast as the problem of estimating the probability that $C = C^r$ for any budget point C^r. Obviously it is pointless to define a subjective probability distribution of C on $[0, C^T]$, but the number of budget points—which equals the number of treatments—is apt to be very small relative to the dollar value of C. For example, the fee schedule for California's Medi-Cal program (the state's name for its Medicaid program) lists roughly 47,000 medical, surgical, and other health care procedures. Treatments in the sense of CEA commonly consist of more than one procedure so that the total number of treatments in a global CEA performed on the Medi-Cal program might be somewhat smaller than 47,000. Suppose, however, the total number of treatments is 47,000. As this is written the annual cost of the Medi-Cal program is approximately $27 billion. Hence for this program the ratio of budget points to total cost is $1/1.7 \times 10^6$, and for any subjective distribution of C on $[0, C^T]$ it is then highly unlikely that C equals any of the budget points C^1 or C^2 or...or C^T.

The issue can be examined from a slightly different angle as well. Suppose it is either known or believed that C is a cost in some budget interval B_{ij}. The length of B_{ij} is $(c_{ij} - c_{ij-1})N_i$. Accordingly, assume that as few as 100 patients have illness i and that the difference in the costs of treatments ij and ij-1 is as little as $10. Even under these extremely conservative assumptions the length of B_{ij} is $1,000, and it can be increased to 100,000 pennies by expressing costs in pennies rather than dollars. Since there are no persuasive reasons for assuming otherwise, it is reasonable for the analyst to think that C is equally likely to be any money value in B_{ij}. Therefore, under these assumptions $Pr[C = C^t | C$ is in $B_{ij}] = 0.001$ if costs are measured in dollars and 0.00001 if they are measured in pennies, and the same kind of reasoning can be applied if it is assumed that C is in one of several or more contiguous budget intervals rather than just one.

At least in the rough ways just described it can be surmised that C is exceedingly unlikely to equal any of the health care agency's budget points. For completeness the condition $C \neq C^t$ will be cited hereafter as a requisite for the validity of the single-treatment GM decision rules, but in performing CEAs on new treatments it is justifiable to ignore the $C \neq C^t$ condition on grounds that it is nearly certainly likely to be satisfied.

Appendix 4   Proof that $R_{h\hat{k}} \leq R_{hm} \leq R_{h\hat{k}+1}$ for all m = k, k+1,..., k*+1 when the new treatment set is of Type 3

First consider the claim that $R_{h\hat{k}} \leq R_{hm}$. It is enough to show that $R_{h\hat{k}} \leq R_{hk}$ when $h\hat{k}$ dominates hk because $R_{hk} \leq R_{hm}$ for each hm by the ordering of the initial treatment set. If $h\hat{k}$ strongly dominates hk, $c_{h\hat{k}} \leq c_{hk}$, $q_{h\hat{k}} \geq q_{hk}$, at least one inequality is strict, and

$$R_{hk} = \frac{c_{hk} - c_{hk-1}}{q_{hk} - q_{hk-1}} > \frac{c_{h\hat{k}} - c_{hk-1}}{q_{h\hat{k}} - q_{hk-1}} = R_{h\hat{k}}.$$

Next, if $h\hat{k}$ and a nondominated treatment hp weakly dominate hk and $c_{h\hat{k}} > c_{hk} > c_{hp}$, $q_{h\hat{k}} > q_{hk} > q_{hp}$, by Lemma 2 and Proposition 2(i),

$$\frac{c_{hk} - c_{hk-1}}{q_{hk} - q_{hk-1}} \geq \frac{c_{hk} - c_{hp}}{q_{hk} - q_{hp}} \geq \frac{c_{h\hat{k}} - c_{hk-1}}{q_{h\hat{k}} - q_{hk-1}},$$

so that

$$(c_{hk} - c_{hk-1})(q_{h\hat{k}} - q_{hk-1} + q_{hk-1} - q_{hk}) \geq (c_{h\hat{k}} - c_{hk-1} + c_{hk-1} - c_{hk})(q_{hk} - q_{hk-1}),$$

and

$$R_{hk} = \frac{c_{hk} - c_{hk-1}}{q_{hk} - q_{hk-1}} \geq \frac{c_{h\hat{k}} - c_{hk-1}}{q_{h\hat{k}} - q_{hk-1}} = R_{h\hat{k}}.$$

122

Hence if $h\hat{k}$ strongly or weakly dominates hk, $R_{h\hat{k}} \leq R_{hm}$.

Now consider the claim that $R_{h\hat{k}+1} \geq R_{hm}$. It is sufficient to show that $R_{h\hat{k}+1} \geq R_{hk^*+1}$ when $h\hat{k}$ dominates hk* because in that case $R_{hk^*+1} > R_{hm}$ for all m < k*. Suppose $h\hat{k}$ strongly dominates hk*. Then $c_{h\hat{k}} \leq c_{hk^*}$, $q_{h\hat{k}} \geq q_{hk^*}$, at least one of inequalities is strict, and

$$R_{hk^*+1} = \frac{c_{hk^*+1} - c_{hk^*}}{q_{hk^*+1} - q_{hk^*}} < \frac{c_{hk^*+1} - c_{h\hat{k}}}{q_{hk^*+1} - q_{h\hat{k}}} = R_{h\hat{k}+1}.$$

Or suppose $h\hat{k}$ and a nondominated treatment hp weakly dominate hk* and $c_{h\hat{k}} > c_{hk^*} > c_{hp}$, $q_{h\hat{k}} > q_{hk^*} > q_{hp}$. By Proposition 2(iii) and Lemma 2 applied to the new treatment set,

$$R_{h\hat{k}+1} = \frac{c_{hk^*+1} - c_{h\hat{k}}}{q_{hk^*+1} - q_{h\hat{k}}} > \frac{c_{h\hat{k}} - c_{hk-1}}{q_{h\hat{k}} - q_{hk-1}} = R_{h\hat{k}} \geq \frac{c_{h\hat{k}} - c_{hp}}{q_{h\hat{k}} - q_{hp}} \geq \frac{c_{h\hat{k}} - c_{hk^*}}{q_{h\hat{k}} - q_{hk^*}}.$$

The inequality between the leftmost and rightmost ICE ratios gives

$$(c_{hk^*+1} - c_{h\hat{k}})(q_{h\hat{k}} - q_{hk^*+1} + q_{hk^*+1} - q_{hk^*}) >$$
$$(c_{h\hat{k}} - c_{hk^*+1} + c_{hk^*+1} - c_{hk^*})(q_{hk^*+1} - q_{h\hat{k}})$$

and

$$R_{h\hat{k}+1} = \frac{c_{hk^*+1} - c_{h\hat{k}}}{q_{hk^*+1} - q_{h\hat{k}}} > \frac{c_{hk^*+1} - c_{hk^*}}{q_{hk^*+1} - q_{hk^*}} = R_{hk^*+1}.$$

Last of all, suppose $h\hat{k}$ and a nondominated treatment hp weakly dominate hk* and $c_{hp} > c_{hk^*} > c_{h\hat{k}}$, $q_{hp} > q_{hk^*} > q_{h\hat{k}}$. By Proposition 2(i) and Lemma 2,

$$\frac{c_{hk^*} - c_{h\hat{k}}}{q_{hk^*} - q_{h\hat{k}}} \geq \frac{c_{hp} - c_{hk^*}}{q_{hp} - q_{hk^*}} \geq \frac{c_{hk^*+1} - c_{hk^*}}{q_{hk^*+1} - q_{hk^*}},$$

and the inequality between the leftmost and rightmost ICE ratios gives

$$(c_{hk^*} - c_{hk^*+1} + c_{hk^*+1} - c_{h\hat{k}})(q_{hk^*} - q_{hk^*+1}) \geq$$
$$(c_{hk^*} - c_{hk^*+1})(q_{hk^*} - q_{hk^*+1} + q_{hk^*+1} - q_{h\hat{k}})$$

and

$$R_{h\hat{k}+1} = \frac{c_{hk^*+1} - c_{h\hat{k}}}{q_{hk^*+1} - q_{h\hat{k}}} \geq \frac{c_{hk^*+1} - c_{hk^*}}{q_{hk^*+1} - q_{hk^*}} = R_{hk^*+1}.$$

Therefore, $R_{h\hat{k}+1} \geq R_{hk^*+1}$ whether $h\hat{k}$ strongly or weakly dominates hk*, and this result completes the demonstration.

5 The Health Care System's Cutoff Point

5.1 The First Concepts and Estimates of the Cutoff Point

Several different concepts of a health care system's cutoff point have been proposed and used in the short history of CEA. If it is assumed the health care agency is a global maximizer its cutoff point is an artifact of its optimizing behavior—maximizing its community's total health benefits subject to a total treatment cost or budget constraint. The system's cutoff point is the marginal cost or producing health benefits at the optimum. It is shown in Chapter 7 that the cutoff point for a myopic optimizer is also the largest marginal cost of health benefits in the health care system, but it cannot be interpreted as a shadow price because the myopic optimizer is not necessarily a global maximizer. Unlike that of the global maximizer, the myopic optimizer's cutoff point can be arbitrarily chosen, but it must still be the largest marginal cost of health benefits in the health care system and it must be realized, not merely proposed, in order for the single-treatment decision rules to become valid.

Neither the GM nor MO health care agency model has been used to rationalize single-treatment CEA. Indeed, until relatively recently no explicit welfare theory has been offered to justify the single-treatment decision rules, and for the most part it appears that analysts and policy makers have regarded the choice of a cutoff point as either arbitrary or self-evident. Nevertheless, during the early 1980s it began to be apparent that the decision rules of CEA as they were then understood were related to the ranking of ICE ratios. Numerical examples suggested that a new or any treatment $h\hat{k}$ could be said to be "cost-effective" if the ICE ratio defined on it and some comparator treatment could be shown to be smaller than the ICE ratio defined on a pair of treatments for at least one other illness. The examples seem to have stimulated the search for the largest of all observed ICE ratios in a health care system—a critical ratio against which $R_{h\hat{k}}$ could be definitively compared—and the search produced empirical rankings of observed ICE ratios that have come to be known as *cost-effectiveness league tables.*

The term "league table" was originally applied to rankings of professional English football teams according to various measures of their athletic performance, but it has also been used in the US and elsewhere to construct performance indicators of institutions such as schools and hospitals. In the 1980s the term was adopted by cost-effectiveness researchers in the UK and US, a few of whom began compiling estimates of the marginal, incremental, or average costs of producing health benefits for treating many different illnesses, the principle data source being published single-treatment CEAs. The largest of the observed or estimated ICE ratios in a cost-effectiveness league table was then taken as the critical ICE ratio for single-treatment CEA—that is, the health care system's cutoff point.

The usefulness of league tables for generating cutoff points in single-treatment CEAs is greatly limited. The data requirements for league tables are so considerable that very few of them have been published, and those that have appeared are mostly out of date (e.g., Drummond et al. [1997], Chapman et al. [2000], Owen et al. [2012]). The older tables could, of course, be updated by inflating treatment prices with a medical care price index, but their usefulness is also impaired by the lack of uniformity of the CEA and other studies from which the ranked ICE ratios are taken. Compilers of league tables have long been criticized for using studies that lack meaningful, comparable definitions and measures of treatment costs, health benefits, or both (e.g., Gerard and Mooney [1993], Mason [1994], Mauskopf et al. [2003], Eichler et al. [2004]), and the largest ICE ratios in published league tables are probably only suggestive of real societal cutoff points. For example, many of the early CEAs used as sources for cost-effectiveness league tables define health benefits as years of life gained from treatments but without adjustments for quality of life. Thus by that definition any treatment that does not extend life—care for simple bone fractures, chronic pain, and non-life-threatening ailments in general—produces zero health benefits. To what extent ignoring the quality-of-life effects of treatments makes for unreliable estimates of ICE ratios and cutoff points is not easy to say, but it is difficult to argue that those estimates are likely to be the same as those obtained with health benefits defined as QALYs.

The second way of specifying cutoff points is an arbitrary one. The best known and most widely employed of these arbitrary cutoff points have been regarded as standards in the US and UK since the turn of the 21st century. The cutoff point for the US health system as a whole is customarily said to be $50,000 per QALY, and for more than a decade the cutoff point for UK's National Health Service has been put at £20,000-£30,000 per QALY by the National Institute for Health and Care Excellence (e.g., Claxton et al. [2002], Devlin and Parkin [2004], Eichler et al. [2004], Evans et al. [2004], Grosse [2008], NICE [2008]). No welfare rationale or other explanation has ever been given for either figure, and although they are still widely used in single-treatment CEAs, they have come to be viewed with skepticism or outright disbelief by many analysts. The origin of the $50,000-per-QALY cutoff point has been described as "murky" (Neumann et al. [2014]), and it is said to have evolved during the course of decisions by the Medicare program in the 1970s or 1980s to insure treatment for end-stage renal disease (Grosse [2008]). The basis for NICE's £20,000-£30,000-per-QALY cutoff point is still more obscure. In the early years in which it was employed NICE even seems to have been reluctant to reveal the value, and it has never said what sort of health welfare performance its cutoff point is intended to achieve. It appears that cost-effectiveness analysts continue to use the arbitrary $50,000-per-QALY and £20,000-£30,000-per-QALY cutoff points only because no other values are currently available.

It has been argued that the $50,000-per-QALY cutoff point in the US is much too low, at least in the sense that it significantly understates the largest observable ICE ratio in the US health care system. Braithwaite et al. [2008]) have estimated the current cost per QALY at as much as $297,000, and raw data also suggest that actual treatment costs are probably substantially greater than $50,000 per QALY. For example, a study of Medicare data for 1991-96 reported an average treatment cost of $37,581 per person during the final year of patients' lives (Hoover et al. [2002]), and updating the average from 1995 to 2015 by the Bureau of Labor Statistics' medical care price index gives a cost of $76,300 per person (US Department of Labor [2015]). Moreover, this updated cost estimate almost certainly greatly understates the largest cost per QALY paid by Medicare. It is unadjusted for quality of life, it does not indicate by how much treatment extended life (at most a year), and it is an average rather than marginal cost of a life-year. For instance, if it is assumed that the average quality of life during the last year is as high as 0.75, the quality-adjusted average treatment cost during the last year of life rises to $101,400.

Still another arbitrary cutoff point has been proposed by the World Health Organization [2014]. It has suggested that each country should set its health care system's cutoff at three times the nation's gross domestic product per capita. In the US in 2015 this dictum would have put the national cutoff point at about $155,000 per QALY (Federal Reserve Bank of St. Louis [2015]). But the proposal comes without a welfare foundation or other justifying argument, and because there is no obvious way of telling what its health care welfare implications are, there seems little reason to accept it. And another problem with this, the $50,000-per-QALY, and any national cutoff point offerings is that they are not agency specific. Unless it can be proved otherwise, it is hard to believe that treatment costs, the distribution of illnesses, or the optimal global patient assignment are the same for all health care agencies—or even all geographic areas—in a nation. For instance, it is not at all evident that the cutoff point for the Medicare program is or should be taken as the same as for all or any of the state Medicaid programs. Furthermore, there may be enough geographic variation in the content and prices of medical treatments to make for differences in global patient assignments even if the communities' medical and health care problems are the same. Insofar as cutoff points can be estimated, it is obviously desirable that they should as much as possible be made agency-specific.

A third method of estimating cutoff points has recently been given by a group of researchers at York University (Claxton et al., [2013]). Primarily, the researchers argue that NICE's £20,000-£30,000-per-QALY cutoff point is one and one-half to nearly two and one-half times as large as it should be, but their work deserves mention mostly for its approach to estimating NICE's (or any agency's) cutoff point. They begin with the normative proposition that the National Health Service should be a global maximizer and that it should seek to maximize its community's total volume of QALYs subject to its budget constraint. They point out correctly that the optimal global patient assignment induces a shadow price of the total cost constraint—the added total cost of producing a QALY—and by econometric methods they go on to estimate this shadow price. However, the immediate difficulty with the approach is that by all accounts the NHS and its research and decision-making arm NICE is not a GM agency, and its global patient assignment is—as the researchers themselves emphasize—not optimal in the GM sense. But the shadow price of the total cost constraint and the agency's cutoff point are meaningful only if they are measured or observed *at the optimum*. In whatever way it is estimated from the NHS's actual non-optimal global patient assignment, the agency's shadow price would equal a GM agency's shadow price of its total cost constraint only by coincidence. To find what a non-GM health care agency's shadow price or cutoff point would be if it were a GM agency, an optimal global assignment must first be estimated or simulated. This requires the estimation of the costs and health benefit products of all treatments for all illnesses, not just those treatments that the NHS actually provides. A point estimate of the optimal marginal cost of health benefits could then be obtained either by applying the prioritization procedure to the set of all treatments or from the optimal solution of the dual linear program described in Chapter 3. The methodology employed by the York University researchers might help NICE or any health care agency reassign its patients to treatments so as to increase its community's total health benefits, but unless it produces an optimal global assignment it cannot find a GM agency's cutoff point.

5.2 Willingness to Pay

The fourth concept of the health care agency's cutoff point began to appear in the CEA literature during the 1990s (O'Brien and Viramontes [1994]), possibly because of what had become the empirical difficulties of establishing a viable largest ICE-ratio cutoff point. As indicated in Chapter 1, it derives from the welfare premise that society has a precise idea of how much it is willing to spend at the margin for health benefits. The premise is known as willingness to pay (WTP), and it holds that a health care agency does or should set a highest price W it is willing to pay for an additional unit of health benefits. This price has the dimensions of an ICE ratio—the added payment made for treatment hk rather than for a less expensive, less health-benefit productive treatment hm, divided by the incremental gain in health benefits produced by hk rather than hm. The largest such price (or marginal cost) W is consequently taken as the health care agency's cutoff point. Presentations and discussions of single-treatment CEA now commonly characterize the health care agency's cutoff point in this way. It is taken as the agency's proper maximum payment for an additional unit of health benefits.

There are two ways of interpreting the use of W in the concept of willingness to pay. The naïve understanding is that W is simply the health care agency's observed cutoff point. In both the GM and MO agency models the cutoff points are the largest marginal costs of health benefits should that the agencies incur. Hence if they are the actual highest marginal costs that the agencies incur, they are the largest incremental payments for health benefits the agencies are observed—and thus presumably willing—to make. Therefore, the GM and MO cutoff points can both be regarded as the revealed maximum prices that the agency acting for its community is willing to pay. But the other interpretation stated in Chapter 1 is normative, that W is the highest price of health benefits that the agency *should* pay. In that sense the WTP premise becomes a welfare axiom opposing Weinstein's Axiom. It is not altogether clear which of these two interpretations, descriptive or normative, is the favored one in the current CEA literature, but it appears to be the latter. For example, a substantial empirical literature now exists on estimates of individuals' willingness to pay for QALYs (e.g., Gyrd-Hansen [2003], Klose [2003], Byrne et al. [2005], King et al. [2005], Lieu et al. [2009], Mason et al. [2009], Bobinac et al. [2010], Shiroiwa et al. [2010], Zhao et al. [2011]). These studies employ a variety of questionnaire, survey, contingent valuation, and other techniques for measuring individual persons' willingness to pay for QALYs. Some of the studies expressly contend or take it as given that their estimates can be used by health care agencies to set ICE-ratio thresholds for CEAs, and for that matter it is hard to see what purpose the results have if they are not intended as estimates of cutoff points for use in CEAs.

The idea that individuals' preferences should determine health care spending appeals to consumer sovereignty, but it does not follow that those preferences, weighed against other expenditure alternatives such as rent or mortgage payments, child care, entertainment, vehicle ownership or leasing, vacation spending, clothing, and the like should determine public expenditures on health care. Presumably W would be chosen by or by agencies created by the community's political institutions—its legislature and executive—and the spending alternatives facing society as a whole, on national defense or domestic law and order, infrastructure, public education, non-health-related welfare, and so forth, are obviously not the same as those facing individuals. The issue of determining willingness to pay is one of public policy, it goes beyond the scope of CEA, and it cannot be resolved by surveys or other investigations of individuals' preferences for receiving health care.

The normative WTP premise is also unrealistic. Government funding authorities do not ordinarily allocate tax and other money resources by setting target marginal costs of the perceived benefits that public programs confer on society, and the WTP premise gives contains no explanation for making public health care spending an exception to the rule. But a theoretical and still more basic flaw in the normative premise is that it makes both total treatment cost and the community's total quantity of health benefits indeterminate. The only criterion for the acceptability of a new or any treatment—that it should be provided to or insured for patients—is that the ICE ratio defined on it and some comparator treatment be no larger than W. Suppose there are $K \geq 2$ treatments for illness h that satisfy this criterion and N_h are patients treated for the illness. Then there are $K \times (N_h+1)$ different single-illness patient assignments for h, $K \times (N_h+1)$ different total costs of treating the illness, and $K \times (N_h+1)$ different quantities of health benefits that patients having the illness receive. The total cost of treating the agency's community is therefore set by W and the way patients distribute themselves among treatments for all illnesses, and there cannot be many governments or health care agencies that do or will allow this sort of result that leaves the total cost of health care unspecified. The health care agency could, of course, select a total cost constraint or have a total cost constraint imposed on it, but in that case there are still $K \times N_h$ different single-illness assignments for h and $K \times N_h$ different quantities of health benefits produced for patients having the illness. Hence by implication and even if it operates with a fixed budget, a WTP health care agency is indifferent to the quantity of health benefits it produces for its patient community, and it is hard to conceive of many such agencies that would willfully behave in that way.

Weinstein's Axiom and the normative WTP premise are competing and contradictory health welfare postulates. Being a global maximizer or an adherent of the WTP premise are not a health care agency's only options, but if the agency is free to pick one or the other, the better choice is the global maximizer model. At any given total cost C a GM agency has exactly one cutoff point $R(C) = R_{ij}$ and produces or has produced exactly one optimal—the largest possible—total quantity of health benefits. Thus If the agency functions with any cutoff point other than $R(C)$, it necessarily obtains a smaller total quantity of health benefits than the optimal quantity. Suppose a WTP agency operates with the same total treatment cost C as a GM agency but with the willingness to pay W chosen as its cutoff point. W is selected exogenously under the normative WTP premise and therefore $W = R(C)$ only by chance. But if $W \neq R(C)$, the WTP agency necessarily produces or has produced a smaller quantity of health benefits than the optimal quantity obtained by the GM agency. Moreover, because the WTP agency's global patient assignment is unspecified, it does not follow that the assignment yields an optimal quantity of health benefits even if $W = R(C)$. Hence pending a proof to the contrary it is reasonable to think that except by chance a WTP agency will produce or have produced a smaller quantity of health benefits than a GM agency. That is, a WTP agency will generally forego—*and be willing to forgo*—some quantity of its community's health benefits in order to sustain its commitment to willingness to pay. Nothing in the normative WTP premise justifies this kind of behavior or explains why a WTP agency should privilege the purported welfare benefits of willingness to pay over the actual health benefits conferred on its community by a GM agency.

Its theoretical and other shortcomings seem sufficient grounds for abandoning the WTP premise in single-treatment CEA. However, in the myopic optimizer model discussed in Chapter 7 it is permitted for the health care agency's cutoff point to be predetermined by an non-optimal initial global patient assignment, and such an assignment can be set by or in conformity with an arbitrary willingness to pay W provided there is an observable ICE ratio R_{hk} = W. A myopic optimizer does not seek a cost-constrained maximum of its community's total health benefits, but it is assumed, given its total cost constraint, to seek the largest possible increase in total health benefits by reassigning patients within a small segment of its health care system. The MO health care agency model is presented on Chapter 7 as a second-best alternative to the global maximizer model when it is reasonable to think that the agency cannot behave as a cost-constrained global maximizer. If for whatever reason a health care agency or the funding or other authority to which the agency is responsible wishes to set the CEA's cutoff point at some observed R_{hk} = W, the MO model is the one to emulate.

5.3 On the Feasibility of Single-Treatment CEA

Even if it is theoretically well-founded, no decision-making procedure is workable if the data it requires are unavailable or of doubtful reliability. In the last two sections it has been argued that the conventional cutoff points of single-treatment CEA have been unreliably estimated or are theoretically unsound, and this raises the natural question of whether single-treatment CEA is empirically workable. The answer is not an unequivocal no, but that the question can be posed is sufficient reason to regard the findings of CEAs with caution. Insofar as it is deemed acceptable to take a conservative approach in evaluating new treatments, it would be helpful to find data or research from which a lower bound on the health care system's cutoff point could be derived. For example, the Medicare end-of-life average treatment costs cited in Section 5.1 might be used if the analysis is to decide whether Medicare should insure the new treatment $h\hat{k}$. Then in a deterministic analysis $h\hat{k}$ could be said conditionally—and conservatively—to be absolutely cost-effective if the

ICE ratio defined on it and the next most costly, most health-benefit productive treatment for h is the largest ICE ratio smaller than this lower bound on the agency's cutoff point. If the ratio is much larger than the lower bound it would be reasonable to conclude that $h\hat{k}$ is not absolutely cost-effective. The strategy's shortcoming is, of course, that it clearly understates the health care system's true cutoff point and thus that it leaves a large element of uncertainty about the true absolute cost-effectiveness of $h\hat{k}$.

As remarked in the preceding chapters, another possibility is to take the cutoff point simply as a parameter of the analysis. In the remaining chapters of the book the agency's cutoff point is nominally regarded as an exogenously set datum, but it is a simple and justifiable matter—and one illustrated in the chapter that follows—to conclude a single-treatment CEA with the statement that $h\hat{k}$ is absolutely cost-effective if and only if the agency's cutoff point is in a critical interval of values. The decision that $h\hat{k}$ is or is not absolutely cost-effective is given to the health care agency and not made by the analyst. The agency is, after all, in a better position than the analyst to know or be able to learn, perhaps with the analyst's assistance, its cutoff point.

If health care agencies could be created as global maximizers it would make the determination of cutoff points a trivial matter. But until that happens or otherwise that the largest ICE-ratio cutoff points are reliably estimated, it should be understood that single-treatment CEAs are useful but as yet imperfect assessors of the desirability of making new treatments available to patients.

References

Bobinac A, van Exel JA, Rutten FFH, Brouwer WBF. Willingness to pay for a quality-adjusted life-year: the individual perspective. Value in Health 2010; 13: 1046-1055

Braithwaite RS, Meltzer DO, King JT Jr, Roberts MS. What does the value of modern medicine say about the $50,000 per quality-adjusted life-year decision rule? Medical Care 2008; 46: 349-56.

Byrne MM, O'Malley K, Suarez-Almazor ME. Willingness to pay per quality-adjusted life year in a study of knee osteoarthritis, Medical Decision Making 2005; 25: 655-666.

Chapman RH, Stone PW, Sandberg EA, Bell C, Neuman PJ. A comprehensive league table of cost-utility ratios and a sub-table of "panel worthy" studies. Medical Decision Making 2000; 20: 638-628.

Claxton, K, Martin S, Soares, M, Rice N, Spackman E, Hinde S, Devlin N, Smith PC, Sculpher M. Methods for the estimation of the NICE Cost Effectiveness Threshold. Final Report. Center for Health Economics, University of York, UK, 2013.

Claxton K, Sculpher M, Drummond M. A rational framework for decision making by the National Institute for Clinical Excellence (NICE). Lancet 2002; 360: 711-715.

Devlin N, Parkin D. Does NICE have a cost-effectiveness threshold and what other factors influence its decisions? A binary choice analysis. Health Economics 2004; 13: 607-639.

Drummond MF, O'Brien B, Stoddart GL, Torrance GW. Methods of Economic Evaluations of Health Care Programmes (2nd ed). Oxford, UK: Oxford University Press, 1997.

Eichler H-G, Kong SX, Gerth WC, Mavros P, Jönsson B. Use of cost-effectiveness analysis in health care resource allocation decision-making: how are cost-effectiveness thresholds expected to emerge? Value in Health 2004; 7: 688-698.

Evans C, Tavakoli M, Crawford B. Use of quality adjusted life years and life years gained as benchmarks in economic evaluations: a critical appraisal. Health Care Management Science 2004; 7: 60-66.

Federal Reserve Bank of St. Louis. Economic Research. Reaearch.stlouisfed.org, 2015.

Gerard K, Mooney G. QALY league tables: handle with care. Health Economics 1993; 2: 59-64.

Grosse SD. Assessing cost-effectiveness in healthcare: history of the $50,000 per QALY threshold. Expert Review of Pharmacoeconomics and Outcomes Research 2008; 8: 165-176.

Hoover DR, Crystal S, Kumar R, Sambamoorthi U, Cantor JC. Medical expenditures during the last year of life: findings from the 1991-1996 Medicare current beneficiary survey. Health Services Research 2002; 6: 1625-42.

King JT, Tsevat J, Lave JR, Roberts MS. Willingness to pay for a quality-adjusted life year: implications for societal health care resource allocation. Medical Decision Making 2005; 25: 667-677.

Klose T. A utility-theoretic model for QALYs and willingness to pay. Health Economics 2003; 12: 17-31.

Lieu TA, Ray GT, Ortega-Sanchez IR, Kleinman K, Rusinak D, Prosser LA. Willingness to pay for a QALY based on community member and patient preferences for temporary health states associated with herpes zoster. Pharmacoeconomics 2009; 27: 1005-1016.

Mason JM. Cost-per-QALY league tables: their role in pharmaco-economic analysis. Pharmacoeconomics 1994; 5: 659-651.

Mauskopf J, Rutten F, Schonfeld W. Cost-effectiveness league tables: valuable guidance for decision makers? Pharmacoeconomics 2003; 21: 991-1000.

National Institute for Health and Care Excellence. Measuring effectiveness and cost effectiveness: the QALY; News report, August 18, 2008. www.nice.org.uk/newsroom/ news/news.jsp.

Neumann PJ, Cohan JD, Weinstein MC. Updating cost-effectiveness—the curious resilience of the $50,000-per-QALY threshold. New England Journal of Medicine 2014; 371, 796-797.

O'Brien B, Viramontes JL. Willingness to pay? A valid and reliable measure of health state preference? Medical Decision Making 1994; 14:289-297.

Owen L et al. The cost-effectiveness of public health interventions. Journal of Public Health 2012; 34, 37-45.

Shiroiwa T, Sung Y-K, Fukuda T, Lang H-C, Bae, S-C, Tsutani K. International survey on willingness-to-pay (WTP) for one additional QALY gained: What is the threshold of cost-effectiveness? Health Economics 2010; 19: 422-437.

US Department of Labor, Bureau of Labor Statistics. www.bls.gov/CPI, 2015.

World Health Organization. Threshold values for intervention cost-effectiveness by region. www.who.int/choice/costs/CERlevels/en/ 2014.

Zhao FL, Yue M, Yang H, Wang T, Wu JH, Li SC. Willingness to pay per quality-adjusted life year: is one threshold enough for decision-making?; results from a study in patients with chronic prostatitis. Medical Care 2011; 49: 267-72.

6 Single-Treatment Cost-effectiveness Analysis in the Global Maximizer Health Care Agency Model: A Summary and Examples

6.1 The Single-Treatment Procedure

The steps in a single-treatment GM CEA are these.

1. Calculate the costs and health benefits of all of the treatments for h including $h\hat{k}$. If this is a particularly onerous task, it may be possible to truncate it by ignoring treatments that are exceptionally expensive or exceptionally ineffective producers of health benefits. The choice of treatments to exclude from the CEA can be left to the analyst, but it should, of course, be made in a responsible fashion and reported to the health care agency.

2. If $c_{h\hat{k}} = c_{hk}$ and $q_{h\hat{k}} = q_{hk}$ for some initial hk (that is, if $h\hat{k}$ is strongly but not strictly dominated by hk), merge $h\hat{k}$ and hk into a single treatment, and relabel the combined treatment $h\hat{k}$. Then using the methods of Chapter 2 remove all other dominated treatments, if there are any, from the treatment set. If $h\hat{k}$ is dominated, it is not absolutely cost-effective for h and the CEA terminates. Otherwise, continue the CEA.

3. Order the remaining treatments in the set so that costs and health benefits per patient increase strictly in the treatment index. By Proposition 3 this can be done when all dominated treatments have been removed from the treatment set.

4. Compute the ICE ratios R_{h2}, $R_{h3}, \ldots,$ $R_{h\hat{k}}, \ldots,$ $R_{hK.}$ that are defined on adjacent treatments in the ordered set. By Proposition 3 the ICE ratios R_{hk} are now ordered so that they increase strictly in the treatment index k. If it is possible to do so, obtain or estimate the health care system's cutoff point R(C). If it is not possible to know or reliably estimate the cutoff point, at the end of the CEA report to the agency the interval of cutoff points for which $h\hat{k}$ is absolutely cost-effective. The agency should know or be able to estimate its own cutoff point, and using rules 5 or 6 below, decide for itself that $h\hat{k}$ is or is not absolutely cost-

effective.

　　5. Determine whether

$$R_{h\hat{k}} = \frac{c_{h\hat{k}} - c_{h\hat{k}-1}}{q_{h\hat{k}} - q_{h\hat{k}-1}} = R(C)$$

or, if there is a treatment $h\hat{k}+1$, whether

$$R_{h\hat{k}+1} = \frac{c_{h\hat{k}+1} - c_{h\hat{k}}}{q_{h\hat{k}+1} - q_{h\hat{k}}} = R(C).$$

If $R_{h\hat{k}} = R(C)$ or $R_{h\hat{k}+1} = R(C)$, declare $h\hat{k}$ to be absolutely cost-effective for h or not as the agency prefers (Proposition 17).

　　6. If $R_{h\hat{k}} \neq R(C)$ and $R_{h\hat{k}+1} \neq R(C)$, apply the maximum ICE-ratio decision rule of Proposition 17. Conclude that $h\hat{k}$ is absolutely cost-effective for h if and only if

$$R_{h\hat{k}} = \max_{m} \{R_{hm} < R(C)\}$$

for all hm in the new treatment set. If $R(C)$ cannot be reliably obtained or estimated, report that $h\hat{k}$ is absolutely cost-effective for h if and only if $R_{h\hat{k}} < R(C) < R_{h\hat{k}+1}$ when there is a treatment $h\hat{k}+1$ and otherwise if and only if $R(C) > R_{h\hat{k}}$.

　　In Chapter 4 it was said that if C equals a budget point, $h\hat{k}$ is not necessarily absolutely cost-effective even though the rules of Proposition 17 imply that it is. The qualification has been omitted in the decision rules presented here for the reason given in Chapter 5 that in any particular CEA the probability that $C = C^t$ for any C^t is almost certainly negligibly small. Nevertheless, if the analyst finds $h\hat{k}$ to be absolutely cost-effective according to the decision rules 5 or 6, she may wish to add the general proviso that the conclusion is conditional on $C \neq C^t$ for all t.

　　Numerical examples of the use of the single-treatment decision rules are presented in the next section. The examples illustrate the use of the rules for various kinds of new treatment sets, and in each example the particular rule's conclusion is verified by performing the prioritization procedure on the agency's global treatment set with $h\hat{k}$ added to it. The examples are intended only as illustrations and they are not meant to represent real-world health care planning scenarios.

6.2. Examples of Single-treatment Global Maximizer CEAs

Consider a small health care agency that cares for a patient community having five illnesses. Initially there are two active treatments each for illnesses 1 and 2, three active treatments each for illnesses 3 and 4, and five active treatments for illness 5. The numbers of patients having the five illnesses are $N_1 = 500$, $N_2 = 400$, $N_3 = 200$, and $N_5 = 300$. The costs and health benefits per treatment of the fifteen active and five no-action treatments for the five illnesses are shown in Table 6.1. In the table the treatments for each illness are ordered so that costs per treatment, health benefits per treatment, and the ICE ratios defined on adjacent treatment pairs all strictly increase in the treatment index. Hence by Proposition 5 there are no dominated treatments in any of the five treatment sets.

If the agency were to use the prioritizing method to find an optimal global patient assignment, it would prioritize the fifteen active treatments as shown in Table 6.2. Table 6.2 is slightly different from Table 3.3 in Chapter 3, where the prioritizing technique is also illustrated because it is intended here to demonstrate how the addition of a new treatment to the global treatment set affects the agency's optimal global assignment.

Suppose the agency's budget or the total cost of the resources it can direct is C = $10.5 million. Then $10.5 million is a cost in the budget interval $(C^{13}, C^{14}] = (\$9.06$ million, $\$10.66$ million], and from Table 6.2 the members of the optimal treatment set are treatments 12, 22, 23, 34, 43, and 56. The health care system's cutoff point is

R($10.5 million) =

$$R_{23} = \frac{C_{23} - C_{22}}{q_{23} - q_{22}} = \$25,000 \text{ per unit of health benefits,}$$

and, although it might not be unobservable to the analyst, illness 2 is the cutoff-point illness. For brevity the units in which ICE ratios are measured

Table 6.1
Treatment Costs, Health Benefits, Incremental Cost-Effectiveness Ratios, and Patient Populations in an Illustrative Health Care System

Treatment	Cost per Treatment in $ (c_{hk})	Health Benefits per Treatment (q_{hk})	ICE Ratio ($ per Benefit)	Patient Population
11	0	0	--	500
12	2,400	0.4	6,000	
13	7,500	0.55	34,000	
21	0	0	--	
22	8,000	1.0	8,000	400
23	12,000	1.16	25,000	
31	0	0	--	
32	250	0.1	2,500	300
33	1,000	0.25	5,000	
34	2,200	0.3	24,000	
41	0	0	--	
42	1,500	0.4	3,750	200
43	5,000	0.75	10,000	
44	18,000	1.25	26,000	
51	0	0	--	300
52	600	3.0	200	
53	2,450	3.5	3,700	
54	5,200	4.0	5,500	
55	6,600	4.2	7,000	
56	10,000	4.4	17,000	

will hereafter be omitted. By Proposition 8 the agency's initial optimal global assignment is:

$$n_{12}(\$10.5 \text{ million}) = 500$$
$$n_{22}(\$10.5 \text{ million}) = 40 = 400 - n_{23}(\$10.5 \text{ million})$$
$$n_{23}(\$10.5 \text{ million}) = 360 =$$

$$(\$10.5\ \text{million} - \$9.06\ \text{million})/(\$12{,}000 - \$8{,}000)$$

$$n_{34}(\$10.5\ \text{million}) = 300$$

$$n_{43}(\$10.5\ \text{million}) = 200$$

$$n_{56}(\$10.5\ \text{million}) = 300$$

all other $n_{hk}(\$10.5\ \text{million}) = 0$.

The initial optimal total quantity of health benefits is 500x0.4 + 40x1.0 + 360x1.16 + 300x0.3 + 200x0.75 + 300x4.4 = 2,217.6 units.

Table 6.2
Initial Prioritized Treatment Set in the Illustrative
Health Care System

t	R_{hk} ($/ Benefit)	Budget Points ($ millions)	Optimal Treatment Set at $C = C^t$	Treatment Enters Optimal Treatment Set at C^{t-1}	Treatment Exits Optimal Treatment Set at C^t
1	--	0	11,21,31,41,51	22	21
2	200	0.18	11,21,31,41,52	52	51
3	2,500	0.255	11,21,32,41,52	32	31
4	3,700	0.81	11,21,32,41,53	53	52
5	3,750	1.11	11,21,32,42,53	42	41
6	5,000	1.335	11,21,33,42,53	33	32
7	5,500	2.16	11,21,33,42,54	54	53
8	6,000	3.36	12,21,33,42,54	12	11
9	7,000	3.78	12,21,33,42,55	55	54
10	8,000	6.98	12,22,33,42,55	22	21
11	10,000	7.68	12,22,33,43,55	43	42
12	17,000	8.70	12,22,33,43,56	56	55
13	24,000	9.06	12,22,34,43,56	34	33
14	**25,000**	10.66	12,23,34,43,56	23	22
15	26,000	13.26	12,23,34,44,56	44	43
16	34,000	15.81	13,23,34,44,56	13	12

C = $10.5 million. Cutoff point in boldface.

Example 1. The initially absolutely cost-effective treatment for illness 3 is treatment 34, but suppose a new treatment 3a becomes available for illness 3 and c_{3a} = $1,800, q_{3a} = 0.29. The treatment set for illness 3 after 3a is added to it is shown in Table 6.3. There are no dominated treatments in the new treatment set because costs and health benefits per treatment and the ICE ratios defined on adjacent treatment pairs all strictly increase in the new treatment index. Furthermore, by inspection of the new treatment set for illness 3, it is evident that neither $(R_{h\hat{k}} =) R_{3a}$ = 15,000 nor $(R_{h\hat{k}+1} =) R_{34}$ = 60,000 equals the health care system's cutoff point. Hence the appropriate decision rule for testing the absolute cost-effectiveness of 3a is the maximum ICE-ratio rule 6. That is, 3a is absolutely cost-effective if and only if

$$R_{3a} = \max_{m} \{R_{3m} < 25{,}000\}.$$

Table 6.3
Example 1. Treatment Costs, Health Benefits, and Incremental Cost-Effectiveness Ratios for the New Treatment Set for Illness 3

Treatment	Cost per Treatment in $ (c_{hk})	Health Benefits per Treatment (q_{hk})	ICE Ratio
31	0	0	--
32	250	0.1	2,500
33	1,000	0.25	5,000
3a	1,800	0.29	20,000
34	2,200	0.3	40,000

By inspection of Table 6.3 is clear that

$$R_{3a} = \max_{m} \{R_{3m} < 25{,}000\}.$$

Thus treatment 3a is absolutely cost-effective for illness 3.

To verify this conclusion, consider the new optimal treatment set obtained by applying the prioritization procedure to the global treatment set after treatment 3a has been added to it. The reprioritized set of all treatments is shown in Table 6.4. The budget interval now containing C is $B_{ij}' = (C^{13}, C^{14}] = (\$8.94$ million,$\$10.54$ million], and everywhere in this interval but at its right endpoint the optimal treatment set is {12, 22, 23, 3a, 43, 56}.

Table 6.4
Example 1. The Prioritized Treatment Set After 3a
Enters the Treatment Set for Illness 3

t	R_{hk} ($/ Benefit)	Budget Points ($ millions)	Optimal Treatment Set at $C = C^t$	Treatment Enters Optimal Treatment Set at C^{t-1}	Treatment Exits Optimal Treatment Set at C^t
1	--	0	11,21,31,41,51		
2	200	0.18	11,21,31,41,52	52	51
3	2,500	0.255	11,21,32,41,52	32	31
4	3,700	0.81	11,21,32,41,53	53	52
5	3,750	1.11	11,21,32,42,53	42	41
6	5,000	1.335	11,21,33,42,53	33	32
7	5,500	2.16	11,21,33,42,54	54	53
8	6,000	3.36	12,21,33,42,54	12	11
9	7,000	3.78	12,21,33,42,55	55	54
10	8,000	6.98	12,22,33,42,55	22	21
11	10,000	7.68	12,22,33,43,55	43	42
12	17,000	8.70	12,22,33,43,56	56	55
13	20,000	8.94	12,22,3a,43,56	3a	33
14	**25,000**	10.54	12,23,3a,43,56	23	22
15	26,000	13.14	12,23,3a,44,56	44	43
16	34,000	15.69	13,23,3a,44,56	13	12
17	40,000	15.81	13,23,34,44,56	34	3a

C = $10.5 million. Cutoff point in boldface.

It is therefore confirmed that 3a is absolutely cost-effective for illness 3. The new optimal global patient assignment—unobservable to

143

the analyst—is

$$n_{12}(\$10.5 \text{ million}) = 500$$
$$n_{22}(\$10.5 \text{ million}) = 10$$
$$n_{23}(\$10.5 \text{ million}) = 390 =$$
$$(\$10.5 \text{ million} - \$8.94 \text{ million})/(\$12,000 - \$8,000)$$
$$n_{3a}(\$10.5 \text{ million}) = 300$$
$$n_{43}(\$10.5 \text{ million}) = 200$$
$$n_{56}(\$10.5 \text{ million}) = 300$$

all other $n_{hk}(\$10.5 \text{ million}) = 0$. The optimal total quantity of health benefits is $500 \times 0.4 + 10 \times 1.0 + 390 \times 1.16 + 300 \times 0.29 + 200 \times 0.75 + 300 \times 4.4 = 2,219.4$ units.

But suppose instead of finding and implementing this optimal global assignment, the agency merely switches all 300 patients having illness 3 from treatment 34 to treatment 3a and leaves the rest of the initial global assignment unchanged. The agency's action reduces its total cost by $\$120,000 = 300 \times (\$2,200 - \$1,800)$ and total health benefits by $3 = 300 \times (0.3 - 0.29)$ units. But the assignment is also optimal at the smaller total cost of $\$10.38$ (= $\$10.5$ million - $\$0.12$ million) because the endpoints of the initial budget interval containing total cost are reduced by the same money value—$\$120,000$—as total cost (see Table 6.4). For example, $n_{23}(\$10.5 \text{ million}) = n_{23}(\$10.38 \text{ million}) = 360 = (\$10.38 \text{ million} - \$8.94 \text{ million})/(\$12,000 - \$8,000)$.

A GM health care agency would *not*, however, choose this optimal global assignment in preference to the optimal global assignment at $C = \$10.5$ million because it leaves $\$120,000$ of idle resources and fails to achieve the largest total quantity of health benefits that could be obtained at $C = \$10.5$ million. In general, when the new absolutely cost-effective treatment is less expensive and less health-benefit productive than the treatment it replaces, a GM health care agency will switch patients from the initially absolutely cost-effective treatment to the new absolutely cost-effective treatment, and *it will revise the initial global assignment* so as to make it optimal at the initial total treatment cost. Failing to do that contradicts Weinstein's Axiom.

Finally, if the analyst is unable to know or estimate health care system's cutoff point, she should report to the agency that 3a

- is not absolutely cost-effective if $R(C) < \$20,000$ per unit of health benefits;
- can be declared absolutely cost-effective or not as the agency prefers if $R(C) = \$20,000$ per unit of health benefits;
- is absolutely cost-effective if $\$20,000 < R(C) < \$40,000$ per unit of health benefits;
- can be declared absolutely cost-effective or not as the agency prefers if $R(C) = \$40,000$ per unit of health benefits; and
- is not absolutely cost-effective for if $R(C) > \$40,000$ per unit of health benefits.

The agency itself must then decide which of these conclusions it should accept, and its decision will depend on what it knows or perceives to be the value of its cutoff point.

Example 2. Again suppose the focal illness is illness 3, but assume the unit cost and health benefit product of the new treatment 3a are $2,800 and 0.32 units respectively. The ordered (by the values of costs and health benefits) treatment set for illness 3 after 3a has been added to it is shown in Table 6.5. Assume as in Example 1 that C = $10.5 million so that the health care system's cutoff point is 25,000. Then 3a neither dominates nor is dominated by other treatments for illness 3, and therefore the appropriate decision rules for the absolute cost-effectiveness of 3a are rules 5 and 6. Since $R_{3a} = 30,000 > R(C) = 25,000$, treatment 3a is not absolutely cost-effective by the maximum ICE-ratio decision rule of step 6. However, if $(R(C)$ were not known, it should be reported that 3a

- is not absolutely cost-effective if $R(C) < 30,000$;
- can be declared absolutely cost-effective or not as the agency

prefers if R(C) = 30,000;

- is absolutely cost-effective if R(C) > 30,000.

Table 6.5

Example 2. Treatment Costs, Health Benefits, and Incremental Cost-Effectiveness Ratios for the Unedited New Treatment Set for Illness 3

Treatment	Cost per Treatment in $ (c_{hk})	Health Benefits per Treatment (q_{hk})	ICE Ratio
31	0	0	--
32	250	0.1	2,500
33	1,000	0.25	5,000
34	2,200	0.3	24,000
3a	2,800	0.32	30,000

To see that 3a is not absolutely cost-effective when as in the example R(C) = 25,000, consider the prioritized global treatment set after 3a has been added to it. The set is shown in Table 6.6. The total cost $10.5 million is a point in the budget interval ($9.06 million,$10.66 million], and the optimal treatment set at all total costs in the interval is {12, 22, 23, 34, 43, 56} except at $10.66 million where treatment 22 is not absolutely cost-effective. Treatment 3a is not a member of this optimal treatment set, and therefore it is not absolutely cost-effective for illness 3 at C = $10.5 million.

Example 3. Assume the initial global treatment set is the same as it is in Example 2, and assume again that the cost and health benefit product of the new treatment 3a are $2,800 and 0.32 units. But now suppose the agency's total treatment cost is $15 million so that the health care system's cutoff point is $34,000. Then by the decision rule 6 treatment 3a is absolutely cost-effective for illness 3 at this total cost, and the correctness of that conclusion can be verified from the prioritized

Table 6.6

Example 2. The Prioritized Treatment Set After 3a Enters the Treatment Set for Illness 3

T	R_{hk} ($/ Benefit)	Budget Points ($ millions)		Treatment Enters Optimal Treatment Set at C^{t-1}	Treatment Exits Optimal Treatment Set at C^t
1	--	0	11,21,31,41,51		
2	200	0.18	11,21,31,41,52	52	51
3	2,500	0.255	11,21,32,41,52	32	31
4	3,700	0.81	11,21,32,41,53	53	52
5	3,750	1.11	11,21,32,42,53	42	41
6	5,000	1.335	11,21,33,42,53	33	32
7	5,500	2.16	11,21,33,42,54	54	53
8	6,000	3.36	12,21,33,42,54	12	11
9	7,000	3.78	12,21,33,42,55	55	54
10	8,000	6.98	12,22,33,42,55	22	21
11	10,000	7.68	12,22,33,43,55	43	42
12	17,000	8.70	12,22,33,43,56	56	55
13	24,000	9.06	12,22,34,43,56	34	33
14	**25,000**	10.66	12,23,34,43,56	23	22
15	26,000	13.26	12,23,34,44,56	44	43
16	30,000	13.44	12,23,3a,44,56	3a	34
17	34,000	15.99	13,23,3a,44,56	13	12

C = $10.5 million. Cutoff point in boldface.

global treatment set shown in Table 6.6. The total treatment cost of $15 million is a point in the budget interval $(C^{16}, C^{17}] = ($13.44$ million, $15.99 million] and except that treatment 12 is excluded at C = $15.99 million, the optimal treatment set at every C in this interval is {12, 13, 23, 3a, 44, 56}. Hence by the prioritization method 3a is absolutely cost-effective for illness 3 at C = $15 million.

Example 4. Assume the initial global treatment set is the one shown in Table 6.1 and as in Examples 1 and 2 that C = $10.5 million and

$R(C) = 25,000$. However, in this example suppose the focal illness is illness 1. Then let 1a be a new treatment for illness 1 costing \$4,900 per patient and producing 0.5 units of health benefits per patient. The new treatment set for illness 1 is shown in Table 6.7, there are no dominated

Table 6.7
Example 4. reatment Costs, Health Benefits, and Incremental Cost-Effectiveness Ratios for the (Edited) New Treatment Set for Illness 1

Treatment	Cost per Treatment in \$ (c_{hk})	Health Benefits per Treatment (q_{hk})	ICE Ratio
11	0	0	--
12	2,400	0.4	6,000
1a	4,900	0.5	25,000
13	7,500	0.55	52,000

treatments in the set, and

$$R_{1a} = \frac{c_{1a} - c_{12}}{q_{1a} - q_{12}} = 25,000 = R(C).$$

Accordingly, by the $R_{h\hat{k}} = R(C)$ decision rule 5 the agency can regard 1a absolutely cost-effective or not as it prefers.

The validity of the $R_{h\hat{k}} = R(C)$ rule in this example is corroborated in Tables 6.8 and 6.9. Illness 2 is the cutoff-point illness i because 23 is the treatment that enters the optimal treatment set at $C = \$10.5$ million (C is in the budget interval (\$9.06 million, \$10.66 million]) and $ij = 23$ (Table 6.6). That is,

$$R_{ij} = R_{23} = \frac{c_{23} - c_{22}}{q_{23} - q_{22}} \text{ is the cutoff point } R(C).$$

Since $R_{1a} = \$25,000$, entering 1a into the treatment set makes it possible to rank R_{1a} higher or lower than R_{23} in the ordered set of all ICE ratios. But the ranking of R_{1a} and R_{23} has no effect on the conclusion that 1a can be declared absolutely cost-effective or not. Tables 6.8 and only

Table 6.8
Example 4. First Prioritized Treatment Set After 1a Enters the Treatment Set for Illness 1

t	R_{hk} ($/ Benefit)	Budget Points ($ millions)	Optimal Treatment Set at $C = C^t$	Treatment Enters Optimal Treatment Set at C^{t-1}	Treatment Exits Optimal Treatment Set at C^t
13	24,000	9.06	12,22,34,43,56	34	33
14	**25,000**	10.31	1a,22,34,43,56	1a	12
15	**25,000**	11.91	1a,23,34,43,56	23	22
16	26,000	14.51	1a,23,34,44,56	44	43
17	52,000	15.81	13,23,34,44,56	13	1a

C = $10.5 million. Cutoff point in boldface.

Table 6.9
Example 4. Second Prioritized Treatment Set After 1a Enters the Treatment Set for Illness 1

t	R_{hk} ($/ Benefit)	Budget Points ($ millions)	Optimal Treatment Set at $C = C^t$	Treatment Enters Optimal Treatment Set at C^{t-1}	Treatment Exits Optimal Treatment Set at C^t
13	24,000	9.06	12,22,34,43,56	34	33
14	**25,000**	10.66	12,23,34,43,56	23	22
15	**25,000**	11.91	1a,23,34,43,56	1a	12
16	26,000	14.51	1a,23,34,44,56	44	43
17	52,000	15.81	13,23,34,44,56	13	1a

C = $10.5 million. Cutoff point in boldface.

6.9 show two prioritized global treatment sets after treatment 1a has entered into it. In Table 6.8, R_{1a} is given the next smaller rank than the rank of R_{23}. In Table 6.9 it is given the next larger rank. Both tables show the bottom five rows of the prioritized treatment arrays—the data associated with the largest five ICE ratios—because rows 1-12 are the same for both arrays.

In Table 6.8 treatment 1a can be seen to be in the optimal treatment set at C > $9.06 million and at all larger costs up to $15.81 million. Thus 1a is optimal at the total cost $10.5 million. But in Table 6.9, 1a enters the optimal treatment set only at C > $10.66 million and remains in the optimal treatment set at all higher total costs < $15.81 million. Therefore, 1a is not absolutely cost-effective for illness 1 at C = $10.5 million. In short, 1a is or is not absolutely cost-effective depending on the arbitrary ranking of R_{1a} and R_{23}. Ranking R_{1a} lower than R_{23} is tantamount to including 1a in the global treatment set, and ranking R_{1a} higher than R_{23} is tantamount to excluding it.

After rounding the numbers of patients to the integer values, by Proposition 8 the optimal global patient assignment for $\rho_{1a} < \rho_{23}$ is, from Table 6.8,

$$n_{1a}(\$10.5 \text{ million}) = 500$$
$$n_{22}(\$10.5 \text{ million}) = 352 = 400 - n_{23}(\$10.5 \text{ million})$$
$$n_{23}(\$10.5 \text{ million}) = 47 =$$
$$(\$10.5 \text{ million} - \$10.31 \text{ million})/(\$12,000 - \$8,000)$$
$$n_{34}(\$10.5 \text{ million}) = 300$$
$$n_{43}(\$10.5 \text{ million}) = 200$$
$$n_{56}(\$10.5 \text{ million}) = 300$$
all other $n_{hk}(\$10.5 \text{ million}) = 0$.

The optimal total quantity of health benefits is 500x.5 + 352.5x1 + 47.5x1.16 + 300x0.3 + 200x0.75 + 300x·4.4 = 2,217.6 units.

For the ranking $\rho_{1a} > \rho_{23}$ the optimal global patient assignment is, from Table 6.9,

$$n_{12}(\$10.5 \text{ million}) = 500$$
$$n_{22}(\$10.5 \text{ million}) = 40 = 400 - n23(\$10.5 \text{ million})$$
$$n_{23}(\$10.5 \text{ million}) = 360 =$$

$$(\$10.5 \text{ million} - \$9.06 \text{ million})/(\$12,000 - \$8,000)$$

$$n_{34}(\$10.5 \text{ million}) = 300$$

$$n_{43}(\$10.5 \text{ million}) = 200$$

$$n_{56}(\$10.5 \text{ million}) = 300$$

all other $n_{hk}(\$10.5 \text{ million}) = 0$,

and, as it was for the first optimal global assignment, the optimal total quantity of health benefits is 500x0.4 + 40x1 + 360x1.16 + 300x0.3 + 200x0.75 + 300x4.4 = 2,217.6 units. As a consequence, each global assignment produces the same total quantity of health benefits, and therefore the agency can declare 1a absolutely cost-effective or not as it prefers with no loss of total health benefits.

Example 5. In Chapter 5 it was said that the GM decision rules can give an incorrect conclusion when $C = C^t$. It can be shown that the rules may be incorrect when $C = C^t$ if in addition

(i) every deleted ICE ratio R_{hm} is smaller than R(C) and

(ii) there are no ICE ratios ranked between R(C) and $R_{h\hat{k}+1}$.

Like the event that $C = C^t$ these two conditions are unobservable to the analyst, but the following example shows their implications when they do occur.

Suppose illness 5 is the focal illness, that 5a is a new treatment for illness 5, and that $c_{5a} = \$7,450$, $q_{5a} = 4.3$. The new ordered treatment set for illness 5 is shown in Table 6.10. Once more let total treatment cost $C = \$10.5$ million so that the cutoff point R($\$10.5$ million) = 25,000. Then the appropriate decision is the maximum ICE-ratio rule 6, and 5a is absolutely cost-effective for illness 5 because $R_{5a} = \$8,500 = \max_{m} \{R_{5m} < 25,000\}$. However, suppose $C = \$10.66$ million instead of $\$10.5$ million. The maximum ICE-ratio decision rule 6 still implies that 5a is absolutely cost-effective for illness 5, but now from Table 6.2 see that C equals the budget point C^{14}. So suppose the global treatment set is reprioritized after 5a is added to it. The reprioritized set is presented in Table 6.11 and it shows that 5a exits the optimal treatment set at $C = \$10.66$ million.

Table 6.10
**Example 5. Treatment Costs, Health Benefits, and Incremental
Cost-Effectiveness Ratios for the First New
Treatment Set for Illness 5**

Treatment	Cost per Treatment in $ (c_{hk})	Health Benefits per Treatment (q_{hk})	ICE Ratio
51	0	0	--
52	600	3	200
53	2,450	3.5	3,700
54	5,200	4	5,500
55	6,600	4.2	7,000
5a	7,450	4.3	8,500
56	10,000	4.4	25,500

Thus at this total cost 5a is not absolutely cost-effective for illness 5. The reasons for the apparent anomaly will be clear. First, in the example only one of the initial ICE ratios defined on of the initial treatments is deleted— the ICE ratio $R_{56} = 17,000$—and this ratio is smaller than the cutoff point 25,000. Second, observe from Table 6.11 that there are no ICE ratios in the new ordered set of all ICE ratios ranked between the cutoff point and the new $R_{56} = 25,500$. Consequently, both of the conditions (i) and (ii) that invalidate the maximum ICE-ratio decision rule when $C = C^t$ are satisfied.

Still, observe that if the data were real it would be an extremely unusual to find that $C = \$10.66$ million. There are 755,000 different dollar values in the budget interval $(C^{14}, C^{15}] = (\$9.85$ million, $\$10.66$ million] that contains total treatment cost, so that the probability that C equals any particular one value such as $\$10.66$ million would generally be negligibly small whatever the distribution of costs in the interval is or is conjectured to be. However, to pursue the example a little further, it can be seen that the maximum ICE-ratio decision rule 6 does give a correct conclusion as to the absolute cost-effectiveness of 5a if the initial $R_{56} < 25,000$ or if

Table 6.11
Example 5. First Reprioritized Treatment Set After 5a Enters the Treatment Set for Illness 5

t	R_{hk} ($/ Benefit)	Budget Points ($ millions)	Optimal Treatment Set at $C = C^t$	Treatment Enters Optimal Treatment Set at C^{t-1}	Treatment Exits Optimal Treatment Set at C^t
1	--	0	11,21,31,41,51		
2	200	0.18	11,21,31,41,52	52	51
3	2,500	0.255	11,21,32,41,52	32	31
4	3,700	0.81	11,21,32,41,53	53	52
5	3,750	1.11	11,21,32,42,53	42	41
6	5,000	1.335	11,21,33,42,53	33	32
7	5,500	2.16	11,21,33,42,54	54	53
8	6,000	3.36	12,21,33,42,54	12	11
9	7,000	3.78	12,21,33,42,55	55	54
10	8,000	6.98	12,22,33,42,55	22	21
11	8,500	7.235	12,22,33,42,5a	5a	55
12	10,000	7.935	12,22,33,43,5a	43	42
13	24,000	8.295	12,22,34,43,5a	34	33
14	**25,000**	9.895	12,23,34,43,5a	23	22
15	25,500	10.66	12,23,34,43,56	56	5a
16	26,000	13.26	12,23,34,44,56	44	43
17	34,000	15.81	13,23,34,44,56	13	12

C = $10.5 million. Cutoff point in boldface.

there exists at least one ICE ratio R_{gm} such that $25,000 \leq R_{gm} \leq$ new R_{56}. For instance, suppose $q_{5a} = 4.2$ as before but $c_{5a} = \$7,350$. With these new values of q_{5a} and c_{5a} the treatment set for illness 5 is shown in Table 6.12. It remains true that

$$R_{5a} = \max_{m} \{R_{5m} < 25,000\}$$

and by the maximum ICE-ratio rule 6 treatment 5a is absolutely cost-

Table 6.12
Example 5. Treatment Costs, Health Benefits, and Incremental
Cost-Effectiveness Ratios for the Second New
Treatment Set for Illness 5

Treatment	Cost per Treatment in $ (c_{hk})	Health Benefits per Treatment (q_{hk})	ICE Ratio
51	0	0	--
52	600	3	200
53	2,450	3.5	3,700
54	5,200	4	5,500
55	6,600	4.2	7,000
5a	7,450	4.3	7,500
56	10,000	4.4	26,500

effective for illness 5 when C = $10.66 million. But now consider the reprioritized global treatment set presented in Table 6.13. The new R_{56} = 26,500 and there exists another ICE ratio R_{44} = 26,000 (see Table 6.1) such that R($10.66 million) = 25,000 < 26,000 < 26,500 = new R_{56}. Accordingly, under these circumstances the maximum ICE-ratio decision rule gives a valid conclusion, and its correctness can be seen by inspection of Table 6.13. Treatment 5a is a member of the optimal treatment set at all C in the interval ($4.005 million, $13.26 million] and it is therefore absolutely cost-effective for illness 5 at C = $10.66 million.

Example 6. In the five examples given above the focal illness is not a cutoff-point illness. The next three examples demonstrate that the decision rules of Proposition 17 are equally applicable when the focal illness is or is perceived to be the cutoff-point illness. Again, it is not necessary for the analyst to know which illness is the cutoff-point illness because the rules of Proposition 17 are not conditional on that knowledge. In these three examples the treatments, population sizes, treatment costs, and treatment health benefits are the same as those in Table 6.1 with one exception. The cost of treatment 44 is assumed to be

Table 6.13

**Example 5. Second Reprioritized Treatment Set After 5a
Enters the Treatment Set for Illness 5**

t	R_{hk} ($/ Benefit)	Budget Points ($ millions)	Optimal Treatment Set at C = C^t	Treatment Enters Optimal Treatment Set at C^{t-1}	Treatment Exits Optimal Treatment Set at C^t
1	--	0	11,21,31,41,51		
2	200	0.18	11,21,31,41,52	52	51
3	2,500	0.255	11,21,32,41,52	32	31
4	3,700	0.81	11,21,32,41,53	53	52
5	3,750	1.11	11,21,32,42,53	42	41
6	5,000	1.335	11,21,33,42,53	33	32
7	5,500	2.16	11,21,33,42,54	54	53
8	6,000	3.36	12,21,33,42,54	12	11
9	7,000	3.78	12,21,33,42,55	55	54
10	7,500	4.005	12,21,33,42,5a	5a	55
11	8,000	7.205	12,22,33,42,5a	22	21
12	10,000	7.905	12,22,33,43,5a	43	42
13	24,000	8.265	12,22,34,43,5a	34	33
14	**25,000**	9.865	12,23,34,43,5a	23	22
15	26,000	12.465	12,23,34,43,5a	44	43
16	26,500	13.26	12,23,34,44,56	56	5a
17	34,000	15.81	13,23,34,44,56	13	12

C = $10.5 million. Cutoff point in boldface.

$17,500 not $18,000. The slightly modified treatment set is displayed in Table 6.14, and the prioritized global treatment set is displayed in Table 6.15. To begin with, suppose C = $12 million. Then by Proposition 8 the initial optimal global patient assignment is

$$n_{12}(\$12 \text{ million}) = 500$$
$$n_{22}(\$12 \text{ million}) = 290 = 400 - n_{23}(\$12 \text{ million})$$

155

Table 6.14

Example 6. Treatment Costs, Health Benefits, Incremental Cost-Effectiveness Ratios, and Patient Populations in an Illustrative Health Care System

Treatment	Cost per Treatment in $ (c_{hk})	Health Benefits per Treatment (q_{hk})	ICE Ratio ($ per Benefit)	Patient Population
11	0	0	--	500
12	2,400	0.4	6,000	
13	7,500	0.55	34,000	
21	0	0	--	
22	8,000	1.0	8,000	400
23	12,000	1.16	25,000	
31	0	0	--	300
32	250	0.1	2,500	
33	1,000	0.25	5,000	
34	2,200	0.3	24,000	
41	0	0	--	200
42	1,500	0.4	3,750	
43	5,000	0.75	10,000	
44	17,500	1.25	25,000	
51	0	0	--	300
52	600	3.0	200	
53	2,450	3.5	3,700	
54	5,200	4.0	5,500	
55	6,600	4.2	7,000	
56	10,000	4.4	17,000	

$$n_{23}(\$12 \text{ million}) = 110 =$$

$$(\$12 \text{ million} - \$11.56 \text{ million})/(\$12,000 - \$8,000)$$

$n_{34}(\$12 \text{ million}) = 300$

$n_{44}(\$12 \text{ million}) = 200$

$n_{56}(\$12 \text{ million}) = 300$

all other $n_{hk}(\$12 \text{ million}) = 0$,

and the initial optimal total quantity of health benefits is 500x0.4 + 290x1.0 + 110x1.16 + 300x0.3 + 200x1.25 + 300x4.4 = 2,277.6 units.

Table 6.15
Example 6. The Initial Prioritized Treatment Set

t	R_{hk} ($/ Benefit)	Budget Points ($ millions)	Optimal Treatment Set at $C = C^t$	Treatment Enters Optimal Treatment Set at C^{t-1}	Treatment Exits Optimal Treatment Set at C^t
1	--	0	11,21,31,41,51	--	--
2	200	0.18	11,21,31,41,52	52	51
3	2,500	0.255	11,21,32,41,52	32	31
4	3,700	0.81	11,21,32,41,53	53	52
5	3,750	1.11	11,21,32,42,53	42	41
6	5,000	1.335	11,21,33,42,53	33	32
7	5,500	2.16	11,21,33,42,54	54	53
8	6,000	3.36	12,21,33,42,54	12	11
9	7,000	3.78	12,21,33,42,55	55	54
10	8,000	6.98	12,22,33,42,55	22	21
11	10,000	7.68	12,22,33,43,55	43	42
12	17,000	8.70	12,22,33,43,56	56	55
13	24,000	9.06	12,22,34,43,56	34	33
14	**25,000**	11.56	12,22,34,44,56	44	43
15	**25,000**	13.16	12,23,34,44,56	23	22
16	34,000	15.71	13,23,34,44,56	13	12

C = $12 million. Cutoff point in boldface.

From Table 6.15, $R_{23} = 25,000$ is the health care system's designated cutoff point and illness 2 is the cutoff-point illness (since $ij = 23$, $ij-1 = 22$, and $n_{43}(\$12\text{million}) = 0$).

Let 4a be a new treatment for illness 4 costing \$1,155 per patient and producing 0.385 units of health benefits. The treatment set for illness 4 after 4a is added to it is shown in Table 6.16, and it is evident from the table that treatment 42 is strictly weakly dominated by treatments 4a and

Table 6.16
Example 6. Treatment Costs, Health Benefits, and Incremental Cost-Effectiveness Ratios for the New Treatment Set for Illness 4 Before It Is Edited

Treatment	Cost per Treatment in \$ (c_{hk})	Health Benefits per Treatment (q_{hk})	ICE Ratio
41	0	0	--
4a	1,155	0.385	3,000
42	1,500	0.40	23,000
43	5,000	0.75	10,000
44	17,500	1.25	25,000

Table 6.17
Example 6. Treatment Costs, Health Benefits, and Incremental Cost-Effectiveness Ratios for the New Treatment Set for Illness 4 After It Is Edited

Treatment	Cost per Treatment in \$ (c_{hk})	Health Benefits per Treatment (q_{hk})	ICE Ratio
41	0	0	--
4a	1,155	0.385	3,000
43	5,000	0.75	10,270
44	17,500	1.25	25,000

43. Therefore, treatment 42 is removed from the treatment set and the new treatment set for illness 4 is shown in Table 6.17. By Inspection of

the table the new treatment set contains no dominated treatments, and $R_{h\hat{k}} = R_{4a} \neq R(\$12 \text{ million})$ and $R_{h\hat{k}+1} = R_{43} \neq R(\$12 \text{ million})$. Thus the appropriate decision rule for the CEA is the maximum ICE-ratio rule 6. By inspection of Table 6.17 $R_{4a} < R_{43} = \max_{m} \{R_{4m} < R(\$12 \text{ million}|4m$ in the new treatment set$\}$, and therefore it should be concluded that 4a is not absolutely cost-effective for illness 4.

The conclusion can be verified by inspection of the new prioritized global treatment set containing 4a that is displayed in Table 6.18.

Table 6.18
Example 6. The Reprioritized Treatment Set After 4a
Enters the Treatment Set for Illness 4

t	R_{hk} ($/ Benefit)	Budget Point ($ millions)	Optimal Treatment Set at $C = C^t$	Treatment Enters Optimal Treatment Set at C^{t-1}	Treatment Exits Optimal Treatment Set at C^t
1		0	11,21,31,41,51	--	--
2	200	0.18	11,21,31,41,52	52	51
3	2,500	0.255	11,21,32,41,52	32	31
4	3,158	0.495	11,21,32,4a,52	4a	41
5	3,700	1.05	11,21,32,4a,53	53	52
6	5,000	1.275	11,21,33,42,53	33	32
7	5,500	2.10	11,21,33,4a,54	54	53
8	6,000	3.30	12,21,33,4a,54	12	11
9	7,000	3.72	12,21,33,4a,55	55	54
10	8,000	6.92	12,22,33,4a,55	22	21
11	10,720	7.68	12,22,33,43,55	43	4a
12	17,000	8.70	12,22,33,43,56	56	55
13	24,000	9.06	12,22,34,43,56	34	33
14	**25,000**	11.56	12,22,34,44,56	44	43
15	**25,000**	13.16	12,23,34,44,56	23	22
16	34,000	15.71	13,23,34,44,56	13	12

C = $12 million. Cutoff point in boldface.

Treatment 4a enters the optimal treatment set at C = $255 thousand and exits at C = $7.68 million. Hence it would be absolutely cost-effective for all total costs larger than $255 thousand and smaller than $7.68 million, but it is not member of the optimal treatment set at the total cost $12 million and at this total cost it is not absolutely cost-effective for illness 4.

Example 7. Assume the global treatment set is the same as that in Example 6 and that C = $12 million, but suppose illness 2 is now the focal illness. From Table 6.15 illness 2 is also the health care system's cutoff-point illness. Let 2a be a new treatment for the illness costing $9,000 per patient and producing 1.1 units of health benefits. The new treatment set for illness 2 is shown in Table 6.19. It is evident from Inspection of the table that the treatment set has no dominated members and that $R_{2a} \neq$ $25,000 = R(C)$. The correct decision rule is therefore the maximum ICE-ratio rule 6, and because

$$R_{2a} = \max_{m} \{R_{2m} < 25,000\}$$

it should be concluded that 2a is absolutely cost-effective for illness 2. The correctness of the conclusion can be verified from the prioritized

Table 6.19
Example 7. Treatment Costs, Health Benefits, and Incremental Cost-Effectiveness Ratios for the New Treatment Set for Illness 2 After 2a Has Been Added to It

Treatment	Cost per Treatment in $ (c_{hk})	Health Benefits per Treatment (q_{hk})	ICE Ratio
21	0	0	--
22	8,000	1.0	8,000
2a	9,000	1.1	10,000
23	12,000	1.16	50,000

global treatment set after 2a has been added to it. The prioritized set is shown in Table 6.20. Notice that to apply the decision rule it is unnecessary to know that illness 2 is the cutoff-point illness. The conclusion is the same whether either illness 2 or illness 4 is taken as the cutoff-point illness. It is only necessary to know that $R_{2a} \neq R(C)$ and $R_{2a+1} \neq R(C)$.

Table 6.20
Example 7. The Prioritized Treatment Set in the Illustrative Health Care System with Treatment 2a Included

T	R_{hk} ($/ Benefit)	Budget Points ($ millions)	Optimal Treatment Set at $C = C^t$	Treatment Enters Optimal Treatment Set at C^{t-1}	Treatment Exits Optimal Treatment Set at C^t
1	--	0	11,21,31,41,51		
2	200	0.18	11,21,31,41,52	52	51
3	2,500	0.255	11,21,32,41,52	32	31
4	3,700	0.81	11,21,32,41,53	53	52
5	3,750	1.11	11,21,32,42,53	42	41
6	5,000	1.335	11,21,33,42,53	33	32
7	5,500	2.16	11,21,33,42,54	54	53
8	6,000	3.36	12,21,33,42,54	12	11
9	7,000	3.78	12,21,33,42,55	55	54
10	8,000	6.98	12,22,33,42,55	22	21
11	10,000	7.38	12,2a,33,42,55	2a	22
12	10,000	8.08	12,2a,33,43,55	43	42
13	17,000	9.1	12,2a,33,43,56	56	55
14	**25,000**	9.46	12,2a,34,43,56	34	33
15	**25,000**	11.96	12,2a,34,44,56	44	43
16	34,000	14.51	13,2a,34,44,56	13	12
17	50,000	15.71	13,22,34,44,56	22	2a

C = $12 million. Cutoff point in boldface.

Example 8. The initial prioritized treatment set is shown in Table 6.15. Let R($12 million) = 25,000 and assume again the focal illness is the cutoff-point illness 2. Now let 2a be a new treatment for illness 2 costing $17,000 per patient and producing 1.36 units of health benefits. The new treatment set for illness 2 is shown in Table 6.21. By inspection of the table it is apparent that treatments 2a and 22 nonstrictly weakly dominate treatment 23, and treatment 23 is therefore removed from the treatment set. The revised new treatment set is shown in Table 6.22.   Now R_{2a} = 25,000 = R($12 million), the appropriate decision rule is rule 5, and 2a can be therefore be declared absolutely cost-effective or not for illness 2 as the health care agency prefers.

Table 6.21
Example 8. Treatment Costs, Health Benefits, and Incremental Cost-Effectiveness Ratios for the New Treatment Set for Illness 2 After 2a Has Been Added to It

Treatment	Cost per Treatment in $ (C_{hk})	Health Benefits per Treatment (q_{hk})	ICE Ratio
21	0	0	--
22	8,000	1.0	8,000
23	12,000	1.16	25,000
2a	17,000	1.36	25,000

Table 6.22
Example 8. Treatment Costs, Health Benefits, and Incremental Cost-Effectiveness Ratios for the New Treatment Set for Illness 2 After 2a Has Been Added and 23 Has Been Deleted

Treatment	Cost per Treatment in $ (C_{hk})	Health Benefits per Treatment (q_{hk})	ICE Ratio
21	0	0	--
22	8,000	1.0	8,000
2a	17,000	1.36	25,000

The prioritized global treatment set with 2a excluded from it is shown in Table 6.15, and the optimal global patient assignment given with Table 6.15 yields an optimal total quantity of health benefits of 2,277.6 units. The prioritized global treatment set including 2a is depicted in Table 6.23, and the optimal global patient assignment associated with the set is, by Proposition 8,

$$n_{12}(\$12 \text{ million}) = 500$$
$$n_{2a}(\$12 \text{ million}) = 48.9 = (\$12 \text{ million} - \$11.56 \text{ million})/$$
$$(\$17,000 - \$8,000)$$
$$n_{23}(\$12 \text{ million}) = 351.1 = (400 - 48.9)$$
$$n_{34}(\$12 \text{ million}) = 300$$
$$n_{44}(\$12 \text{ million}) = 200$$
$$n_{56}(\$12 \text{ million}) = 300$$
all other $n_{hk}(\$12 \text{ million}) = 0$.

The optimal total quantity of health benefits produced by the assignment is 500x0.4 + 48.9x1.36 + 351.1x1.0 + 300x0.3 + 200x1.25 + 300x4.4 = 2,277.6 units. Thus the agency can declare 2a absolutely cost-effective or not and assign patients to either treatment 2a or treatment 23 with no loss of health benefits at C = $12 million.

Because of the arbitrary ranking of R_{23} and R_{44}—$\rho_{44} < \rho_{23}$—n the initial prioritized global treatment set (Table 6.15), it might be thought that this conclusion can change if the ranking were to be reversed and illness 4 is made the cutoff-point illness. But that is not the case. Suppose $\rho_{23} < \rho_{44}$. The prioritized initial global treatment set—excluding treatment 2a—with this ranking of treatments 23 and 44 is shown in Table 6.24, the new optimal global patient assignment is

$$n_{12}(\$12 \text{ million}) = 500$$
$$n_{23}(\$12 \text{ million}) = 400$$
$$n_{34}(\$12 \text{million}) = 300$$
$$n_{43}(\$12 \text{ million}) = 200 - 107.2 = 92.8$$
$$n_{44}(\$12 \text{ million}) =$$

$$(\$12 \text{ million} - \$10.66 \text{ million})/(\$12{,}500) = 107.2$$

$$n_{56}(\$12 \text{ million}) = 300$$

all other $n_{hk}(\$12 \text{ million}) = 0$,

and the optimal total quantity of health benefits is 500x0.4 + 400x1.16 + 300x0.3 + 92.8x0.75 + 107.2x1.25 + 300x4.4 = 2,277.6 units.

Table 6.23
Example 8. The Prioritized Treatment Set in the Illustrative Health Care System with Treatment 2a Included

t	R_{hk} ($/ Benefit)	Budget Points ($ millions)	Optimal Treatment Set at $C = C^t$	Treatment Enters Optimal Treatment Set at C^{t-1}	Treatment Exits Optimal Treatment Set at C^t
1	--	0	11,21,31,41,51		
2	200	0.18	11,21,31,41,52	52	51
3	2,500	0.255	11,21,32,41,52	32	31
4	3,700	0.81	11,21,32,41,53	53	52
5	3,750	1.11	11,21,32,42,53	42	41
6	5,000	1.335	11,21,33,42,53	33	32
7	5,500	2.16	11,21,33,42,54	54	53
8	6,000	3.36	12,21,33,42,54	12	11
9	7,000	3.78	12,21,33,42,55	55	54
10	8,000	6.98	12,22,33,42,55	22	21
11	10,000	7.68	12,22,33,43,55	43	42
12	17,000	8.70	12,22,33,43,56	56	55
13	24,000	9.06	12,22,34,43,56	34	33
14	**25,000**	11.56	12,22,34,44,56	44	43
15	**25,000**	15.16	12,2a,34,44,56	2a	22
16	34,000	17.71	13,2a,34,44,56	13	12

C = $12 million. Cutoff point in boldface.

Table 6.24

Example 8. The Initial Prioritized Treatment Set with $\rho_{23} < \rho_{44}$

t	R_{hk} ($/Benefit)	Budget Points ($ millions)	Optimal Treatment Set at $C = C^t$	Treatment Enters Optimal Treatment Set at C^{t-1}	Treatment Exits Optimal Treatment Set at C^t
1	--	0	11,21,31,41,51	--	--
2	200	0.18	11,21,31,41,52	52	51
3	2,500	0.255	11,21,32,41,52	32	31
4	3,700	0.81	11,21,32,41,53	53	52
5	3,750	1.11	11,21,32,42,53	42	41
6	5,000	1.335	11,21,33,42,53	33	32
7	5,500	2.16	11,21,33,42,54	54	53
8	6,000	3.36	12,21,33,42,54	12	11
9	7,000	3.78	12,21,33,42,55	55	54
10	8,000	6.98	12,22,33,42,55	22	21
11	10,000	7.68	12,22,33,43,55	43	42
12	17,000	8.70	12,22,33,43,56	56	55
13	24,000	9.06	12,22,34,43,56	34	33
14	**25,000**	10.66	12,23,34,43,56	23	22
15	**25,000**	13.16	12,23,34,44,56	44	43
16	34,000	15.71	13,23,34,44,56	13	12

C = $12 million. Cutoff point in boldface.

The prioritized global treatment set including treatment 2a and excluding treatment 23 is shown in Table 6.25, and with this ranking of R_{2a} and R_{44} the optimal global patient assignment is

$$n_{12}(\$12 \text{ million}) = 500$$
$$n_{22}(\$12 \text{ million}) = 73.3 = 400 - n_{2a}(\$12 \text{ million})$$
$$n_{2a}(\$12 \text{ million}) = 326.7 = (\$12,000,000 - \$9,060,000)/$$
$$(\$17,000 - \$8,000)$$
$$n_{34}(\$12 \text{ million}) = 300$$
$$n_{44}(\$12 \text{ million}) = 200$$

$n_{56}(\$12 \text{ million}) = 300,$

all other $n_{hk}(\$12 \text{ million}) = 0.$

Table 6.25

Example 8. The Prioritized Treatment Set in the Illustrative Health Care System with Treatment 2a Included and $\rho_{2a} < \rho_{44}$

t	R_{hk} ($/ Benefit)	Budget Points ($ millions)	Optimal Treatment Set at C = C^t	Treatment Enters Optimal Treatment Set at C^{t-1}	Treatment Exits Optimal Treatment Set at C^t
1	--	0	11,21,31,41,51		
2	200	0.18	11,21,31,41,52	52	51
3	2,500	0.255	11,21,32,41,52	32	31
4	3,700	0.81	11,21,32,41,53	53	52
5	3,750	1.11	11,21,32,42,53	42	41
6	5,000	1.335	11,21,33,42,53	33	32
7	5,500	2.16	11,21,33,42,54	54	53
8	6,000	3.36	12,21,33,42,54	12	11
9	7,000	3.78	12,21,33,42,55	55	54
10	8,000	6.98	12,22,33,42,55	22	21
11	10,000	7.68	12,22,33,43,55	43	42
12	17,000	8.70	12,22,33,43,56	56	55
13	24,000	9.06	12,22,34,43,56	34	33
14	**25,000**	12.66	12,2a,34,43,56	2a	22
15	**25,000**	15.16	12,2a,34,44,56	44	43
16	34,000	17.71	13,2a,34,44,56	13	12

C = $12 million. Cutoff point in boldface.

The optimal total quantity of health benefits is 500x0.4 + 73.3x1.0 + 326.7x1.36 + 300x0.3 + 200x0.75 = 2,277.6 units. Thus it makes no difference whether illness 4 or illness 2 is designated the cutoff-point illness. The decision rule's conclusion is the same for each of the rankings of 23 and 44. At C = $12 million treatment 2a is optimal when 23 is excluded from the treatment set for illness 2, and treatment 23 is optimal when 2a is excluded from the set. Moreover, each optimal global patient assignment produces the same total quantity of health benefits.

6.3 Managing the Health Care System When a New Treatment Is Found to Be Absolutely Cost-Effective

The salient feature of single-treatment CEA—and explicit in the GM model—is that the health care agency deploys its resources as best it can to produce the largest total quantity of health benefits for its patients. In practice it would seem a trivial matter to follow this principle. However, it was mentioned in Chapter 1 that the UK's National Institute for Health and Care Excellence is said to accept putatively cost-effective but expensive new treatments and the National Health Service then increases its total cost in order to provide them to patients. Insofar as there exists a tendency for health care agencies to act in this way—to decide that new treatments are cost-effective and then increase their total costs as necessary to provide or insure the treatments for patients—it nullifies the welfare purpose of CEA. A new treatment is provably absolutely cost-effective only at the agency's initial total cost. The GM agency's optimal treatment set changes with its total treatment cost, and when its treatment cost is allowed to increase, the new treatment may or may not still be absolutely cost-effective at the higher total cost. A second single-treatment CEA must be performed in order to be sure that the new treatment is absolutely cost-effective at the new total cost.

Nor, if offering a new absolutely cost-effective treatment to patients increases both total health benefits and total treatment cost, does the result necessarily improve the community's overall wellbeing. Increasing expenditure on health care draws resources away from other public programs, and the issue then is whether this expenditure might better be made on those other programs than on health care. The question of how public funds should be allocated for health care and non-health-care goods and services falls outside the scope of CEA, but the allocative problem needs to be recognized when decisions are made about how to implement the conclusions of CEAs. It is convenient but wrong for a health care agency to think that its work is done when after judging a new treatment to be absolutely cost-effective, it needs only to sanction the treatment for its patients. To make sure that providing or insuring a new absolutely cost-effective treatment increases the community's health wellbeing without reducing the community's non-health-related welfare, the agency must maintain a fixed total treatment cost. Thus each time the agency adds an absolutely cost-effective treatment to its set of all treatments for its patients it must usually find and put into effect a new optimal global assignment at its initial total treatment cost.

7 Deterministic Single-Treatment Cost-Effectiveness Analysis in the Myopic Optimizer Model: the Decision Rules

7.1 Introduction

The appeal of the global maximizer model of CEA is twofold. First, it provides a unified theory of CEA. The global and single-treatment decision rules can be deduced from the same model of a health care agency's behavior, and the single-treatment rules can be derived, albeit with some effort, from the global rules. It is unnecessary to think of the global and single-treatment forms of CEA as unconnected and having possibly different welfare implications for the agency's community. The second attractive feature of the GM model it its explicit utilitarian welfare foundation. The utilitarian ethic of GM CEA is not the only welfare principle used in or recommended for public policy, but in many instances it is deemed an acceptable one, and if the health care agency, its community, or health care policy makers believe otherwise they have the choice of rejecting both it and Weinstein's Axiom.

It can be questioned, though, whether the GM model is a realistic one, whether health care agencies typically or usually behave as GM agencies even if they nominally endorse Weinstein's Axiom. An agency may be unable or unwilling to revise its global patient assignment in response to frequent changes in its treatment offerings, treatment costs, or treatment effectiveness for any of a variety of reasons. The cost of the revisions may be substantial, the agency's management may be understaffed, inexperienced, or otherwise inefficient, or there might be resistance to change from providers or patients. But because the single-treatment decision rules are derived from the premise that the agency maximizes total health benefits given its total cost, they may seem to lose their foundation and relevance if the agency does not rigorously pursue this cost-constrained maximum or pursues it but does not rigorously achieve it. This chapter therefore presents a variant of the GM model that yields single-treatment decision rules that are in essence identical to those of the GM model but in which the agency does not necessarily seek or attain a cost-constrained maximum of total health benefits.

An organization that is a myopic optimizer seeks to optimize a global objective function defined on an engineering, economic, financial, or other system but is unable to achieve a global optimum because it lacks full knowledge of or control over the system's global behavior. Instead, the myopic optimizer attempts to improve the overall performance of its system incrementally by acting on and managing only that component of the system that it does understand and can control. In effect, the manager either chooses to act or is forced to act short-sightedly. It "sees" only a small portion of the large system and ignores what it cannot "see". Operationally, it is confronted by an event of some kind that changes or may change the system's performance, and it responds to this event by finding and effectuating an action that brings about the largest possible increase in its objective function. The myopic optimum may or may not be a global optimum, but its value is the largest the manager can obtain given its limited information or limited ability to control its global system.

So that it has a name the variant of the GM model discussed in this chapter will be called the *myopic optimizer* (MO) model. In the model it is assumed that the health care agency is faced with the same single-treatment decision as the GM agency—whether to provide or sanction a new treatment for some focal illness. The introduction of the new treatment is an event that, if the agency acts on it, changes or may change the quantity of health benefits produced by the health care system. The availability of the new treatment presents the agency with the opportunity to revise its patient assignment for the focal illness so as to increase total health benefits. The MO agency's objective function is, like the GM agency's, the community's total health benefits expressed as a function of total cost, but unlike the GM agency the MO agency does not necessarily seek a cost-constrained global maximum of total health benefits.

One kind of myopic optimizing procedure for deciding the absolute cost-effectiveness of new treatments consists of finding the patient assignment for the focal illness that maximizes the total health benefits of patients having the illness without changing the initial total cost of treating the illness. A new treatment is then absolutely cost-effective for the illness if and only if in the cost-constrained health-benefits maximizing patient assignment a positive number of patients is assigned to the new treatment. The optimization procedure is a simple one and its details will be left to the reader. The procedure does, however, have its limitations for health care policy, a practical one of which is that it requires the analyst to know the initial total cost of caring for the focal illness h. Determining this cost is not impossible—it could be deduced from the agency's claims records or estimated as the sum of the products $c_{hk}n_{hk}$ from the agency's initial assignment to h—but both of these methods necessitate the use of information not ordinarily available to analysts. In addition, the options for increasing the community's total health benefits are restricted to the opportunities available by revising the assignment to only one illness. If the options were extended to revisions of the assignments to h and to other illnesses as well, the increase in the community's total health benefits could not be smaller than the increase obtainable from a revision of the assignment to h and it could be larger. In any event, the one-illness maximization procedure for deciding absolute cost-effectiveness is mentioned as an alternative for health care agencies and health care policy makers to consider, but it will not be discussed in this book.

Instead, another and more general procedure will be presented that does not restrict patient reassignment possibilities to patients having only the focal illness. This procedure is followed by a model MO agency that, when a new treatment $h\hat{k}$ for illness h becomes available:

(i) chooses an assignment for h and perhaps one or a few other illnesses that yields the largest increase in the health care system's total health benefits without changing its total cost; but

(ii) makes no other revisions in its initial global assignment. This new assignment to treatments for h is myopically optimal.

(iii) The new treatment $h\hat{k}$ is then to be offered to patients having h if and only if the number of patients $n_{h\hat{k}}$ assigned to $h\hat{k}$ is positive.

(The definition of "a few other illnesses" is left unspecified except that it implies that the agency does not attempt to revise its entire global patient assignment.) To carry out this procedure it will be assumed that the analyst has the same information as the GM analyst, namely that she knows or has or accurate estimates of:

(i) the costs and health benefit products of all treatments for the focal illness, and

(ii) the health care system's cutoff point.

Two types of cost-effectiveness, relative and absolute, were defined for the GM model. In this chapter the same two types of cost-effectiveness will be used for the MO model but their meanings will be slightly rephrased. The first definition is this.

Definition. Assume a global assignment in which the numbers of patients assigned to two treatments hk and $h\hat{k}$ for illness h are $n_{hk} > 0$ and $n_{h\hat{k}} \geq 0$. Then $h\hat{k}$ is cost-effective relative to hk if there exists another global assignment in which one or more patients are switched from hk to $h\hat{k}$, total health benefits are at least as large as the quantity produced by the initial global assignment, and total cost is unchanged or reduced.

Observe that if $h\hat{k}$ is not cost-effective relative to hk, hk is cost-effective relative to $h\hat{k}$. Also notice that having the property of relative cost-effectiveness is transitive—i.e., if hk is cost-effective relative to hm and $h\hat{k}$ is cost-effective relative to hk, $h\hat{k}$ is cost-effective relative to hm.

More specifically, if with total treatment cost fixed total health benefits can be increased or not changed by switching patients from $h\hat{k}$ to hk and also from hk to hm, then total health benefits can be increased or not reduced by switching patients directly from $h\hat{k}$ to hm.

The definition of absolute cost-effectiveness for the MO model is now this:

Definition. A treatment $h\hat{k}$ is absolutely cost-effective (myopically optimal) for illness h if it is cost-effective relative to every other treatment for h.

Thus treatment $h\hat{k}$ is absolutely cost-effective for h, if with total treatment cost fixed, it is not possible to switch patients from $h\hat{k}$ to any other treatment for h and thereby increase total health benefits. Reassigning patients to $h\hat{k}$ from hk with total cost constant therefore yields the largest provable increase in total health benefits with respect to the agency's initial quantity of health benefits. *Accordingly, $h\hat{k}$ should be provided to or sanctioned for patients if and only if it is absolutely cost-effective for h.*

As it is for a GM agency, a strictly dominated treatment cannot be absolutely cost-effective because it is not cost-effective relative to the treatment or treatments that dominate it. But switching patients from any dominated treatment to the dominating treatment(s) does not increase total health benefits with total cost constant or does not reduce total cost with total health benefits constant. As a consequence, there are never advantages in providing or insuring a dominated treatment in place of the dominating treatment(s), and with one exception dominated treatments will therefore never be considered absolutely cost-effective. The exception is again the case in which two or more treatments nonstrictly strongly dominate one another. If $c_{hk} = c_{hm}$ and $q_{hk} = q_{hm}$, hk and hm are identical for the purposes of CEA and they will be merged into a single treatment. As before, if the composite treatment is found to be absolutely cost-effective, the health care agency can assign patients to the composite's components in any way it prefers. There is no exception, however, for nonstrictly weakly dominated treatments. As was said in Chapter 2, it is not possible to merge a nonstrictly weakly dominated treatment with the two dominating treatments and distribute patients arbitrarily among the three treatments so as to define a fixed cost a fixed quantity of health benefits of the composite treatment. Hence it will be assumed that all dominated treatments except those that are nonstrictly strongly dominated and merged into composites are deleted from the set for treatments for the focal illness during a single-treatment MO CEA. Alternatively, if two or more treatments nonstrictly strongly dominate one another, the agency can, if it prefers to do so, delete one of them from the treatment set. Whether or not the agency takes this second option, the new edited treatment set for h—containing $h\hat{k}$—will always have no dominated members.

Testing the cost-effectiveness of $h\hat{k}$ relative to another treatment hk for h entails three steps:

(i) hypothetically switching patients from hk to $h\hat{k}$;

(ii) hypothetically switching other patients among other treatments to offset the change in costs caused by the first reassignment; and

(iii) measuring the resulting change in health benefits.

To conduct the analysis it must be assumed in that patients can be switched to $h\hat{k}$ from every other treatment for illness h—i.e., that initially $n_{hk} > 0$ for all hk. A real MO health care agency may not assign patients to each of the initial treatments for h, but if $h\hat{k}$ is not cost-effective relative to all of the other treatments for h, it is not absolutely cost-effective for the illness. Thus regardless of the actual number of initial treatments to which patients are assigned, the analyst must test the cost-effectiveness of $h\hat{k}$ relative to every other treatment for h. And to do that it must be supposed that patients can be reassigned to $h\hat{k}$ from every other treatment hk for illness h whether or not $n_{hk} = 0$. By this supposition it can be decided that h$\hat{\text{k}}$ is or is not cost-effective relative to each of the other treatments for h whatever the agency's initial assignment to h is.

The health care system's cutoff point is defined as it is in the GM model, which is to say it is the largest ICE ratio—the largest observable marginal cost of producing health benefits—measured on treatment pairs in the health care system. The ratio is defined on two treatments for some illness i, and i then becomes the cutoff-point illness. The MO cutoff point will be denoted R(A) where A stands generically for the agency's name or identity. In general the MO cutoff point R(A) will vary from agency to agency even if patient populations, the global set of treatments, total treatment costs, and individual treatment costs and health benefits are the same. But to make the definition of the cutoff point specific, consider all illnesses g such that the agency assigns patients to at least two treatments for each of them. For each illness g consider both the costliest, most health-benefit productive treatment gp and the second costliest, most health-benefit productive treatment gp' to which positive numbers of patients are assigned. Then the ICE ratio

$$\frac{c_{gp} - c_{gp'}}{q_{gp} - q_{gp'}}$$

is observable, the cutoff point is defined as

$$R(A) = \frac{c_{ij} - c_{ij'}}{q_{ij} - q_{ij'}} = \max_{\text{all } g} \left\{ \frac{c_{gp} - c_{gp'}}{q_{qp} - q_{qp'}} \right\},$$

and R(A) is therefore observable as well. Although illness i is the cutoff-point illness, gp' is not—as it is for a GM agency—necessarily the second costliest, most health-benefit productive treatment for gp. It may be that gp" is that treatment but that the agency does not assign a positive number of patients to gp".

As was done for the GM agency model it will be assumed that R(A) is a given datum, but if there is no R(A) satisfying the defining criteria or the estimate of R(A) is deemed unreliable, the cutoff point should be taken as a parameter of the analysis. Then the conclusion of the CEA should state that $h\hat{k}$ is or can be declared absolutely cost-effective for illness h if and only if R(A) is an ICE ratio in a particular interval of values determined by the analysis. Observe that when an observable R(A) is accepted as the MO agency's cutoff point, it will not generally be the same as the GM cutoff point R(C) even if the global treatment cost are the same set are exactly the same for both agencies. The MO agency does not necessarily maintain an optimal global patient assignment, and insofar as it does not, the treatments to which it assigns patients and its cutoff point will not be the same as those of a GM agency.

The next section states and proves the basic rules for deciding the absolute cost-effectiveness of $h\hat{k}$ for the focal illness. As in the GM model it is assumed that all costs are direct and that the costs and health benefits of no-action treatments are zero.

7.2 Rules for Deciding the Absolute Cost-Effectiveness of a New Treatment $h\hat{k}$

Treatment $h\hat{k}$ is cost-effective relative to another treatment hk if it is possible to switch patients from hk to $h\hat{k}$ and to switch other patients between treatments for h or a small number of other illnesses so as to increase or not reduce total health benefits without increasing total cost. With the information assumed available to her, the MO analyst is always able to prove that patients can be reassigned from hk to $h\hat{k}$ so as to keep total cost unchanged, and then the only issue is whether the reassignment increases or does not reduce total health benefits.

The decision rules for a single-treatment MO CEA are the same as those for a single-treatment GM CEA. After all nonstrictly strongly dominated treatments in the new treatment set are combined, the only strongly dominated remaining members of the set are strictly dominated. And because $h\hat{k}$ is always cost-effective relative to an hk if it strongly dominates hk, hk is then removed from the set. The other necessary and sufficient conditions for the relative cost-effectiveness of $h\hat{k}$ when it does not dominate hk are given in Propositions 18 and 19. Necessary and sufficient conditions for the absolute cost-effectiveness of $h\hat{k}$ are given by Propositions 20 and 21.

Proposition 18. Let $h\hat{k}$ be added to the treatment for illness h and assume that $h\hat{k}$ does not strongly dominate and is not strongly dominated by another treatment hk. Then when $c_{h\hat{k}} > c_{hk}$ and $q_{h\hat{k}} > q_{hk}$, $h\hat{k}$ is cost-effective relative to hk if and only if

$$\frac{c_{h\hat{k}} - c_{hk}}{q_{h\hat{k}} - q_{hk}} \leq R(A).$$

Treatments $h\hat{k}$ and hk are cost-effective relative to one another if and only if

$$\frac{c_{h\hat{k}} - c_{hk}}{q_{h\hat{k}} - q_{hk}} = R(A),$$

and, given total cost, total health benefits are the same whether patients are assigned to $h\hat{k}$ or hk.

Proof: Because $h\hat{k}$ does not strongly dominate and is not strongly dominated by hk, it must be either that $c_{h\hat{k}} > c_{hk}$ and $q_{h\hat{k}} > q_{hk}$ or that $c_{h\hat{k}} < c_{hk}$ and $q_{h\hat{k}} < q_{hk}$. Assume that $c_{h\hat{k}} > c_{hk}$ and $q_{h\hat{k}} > q_{hk}$ and suppose also that

$$\frac{c_{h\hat{k}} - c_{hk}}{q_{h\hat{k}} - q_{hk}} \leq R(A).$$

Then there exists at least one pair of treatments gp and gp' such that $c_{gp} > c_{gp'}$, $q_{gp} > q_{gp'}$, $n_{gp} > 0$, and

$$R(A) \geq \frac{c_{gp} - c_{gp'}}{q_{gp} - q_{gp'}} \geq \frac{c_{h\hat{k}} - c_{hk}}{q_{h\hat{k}} - q_{hk}}.$$

(For example, let gp = ij and gp' = ij'.) Let Δn_h patients be reassigned from hk to $h\hat{k}$ and Δn_g patients be reassigned from gp to gp' so that $\Delta n_h(c_{h\hat{k}} - c_{hk}) - \Delta n_g(c_{gp} - c_{gp'}) = 0$. Then total cost is unchanged,

$$\frac{\Delta n_h (c_{h\hat{k}} - c_{hk})}{\Delta n_h (q_{h\hat{k}} - q_{hk})} \leq \frac{\Delta n_g (c_{gp} - c_{gp'})}{\Delta n_g (q_{gp} - q_{gp'})} = \frac{\Delta n_h (c_{h\hat{k}} - c_{hk})}{\Delta n_g (q_{gp} - q_{gp'})},$$

and the net change in total health benefits is $\Delta n_h (q_{h\hat{k}} - q_{hk})$ - $\Delta n_g (q_{gp} - q_{gp'}) \geq 0$, with equality if and only if

$$\frac{c_{h\hat{k}} - c_{hk}}{q_{h\hat{k}} - q_{hk}} = R(A).$$

Therefore, there exists at least one new global assignment that yields as large a quantity of total health benefits as the initial global assignment and at the same total cost. Hence $h\hat{k}$ and hk are cost-effective relative to one another if

$$\frac{c_{h\hat{k}} - c_{hk}}{q_{h\hat{k}} - q_{hk}} = R(A) = \frac{c_{ij} - c_{ij'}}{q_{ij} - q_{ij'}}$$

Moreover, since $\Delta n_h (q_{h\hat{k}} - q_{hk})$ - $\Delta n_g (q_{gp} - q_{gp'}) = 0$ if and only if

$$\frac{c_{h\hat{k}} - c_{hk}}{q_{h\hat{k}} - q_{hk}} = R(A),$$

total health benefits are unchanged when patients are switched from hk to $h\hat{k}$—and back from $h\hat{k}$ to hk.

Suppose now that $h\hat{k}$ is cost-effective relative to hk. Then it must be possible to switch patients from hk to $h\hat{k}$ and from some more expensive treatment for another illness to a less expensive treatment for that same illness so as to preserve the constancy of total cost and increase or not reduce total health benefits. Treatments gp and gp' are candidates for this second pair of treatments. Accordingly, switch Δn_h patients from hk to $h\hat{k}$ and Δn_g patients from gp to gp' so that $\Delta n_h (c_{h\hat{k}} - c_{hk})$ - $\Delta n_g (c_{pg} - c_{pg'}) = 0$. Moreover, it must also be true that $\Delta n_h (q_{h\hat{k}} - q_{hk})$ - $\Delta n_g (q_{qp} - q_{qp'}) \geq 0$. Therefore,

$$\frac{c_{h\hat{k}} - c_{hk}}{q_{h\hat{k}} - q_{hk}} = \frac{\Delta n_h (c_{h\hat{k}} - c_{hk})}{\Delta n_h (q_{h\hat{k}} - q_{hk})} \leq \frac{\Delta n_h (c_{h\hat{k}} - c_{hk})}{\Delta n_g (q_{gp} - q_{gp'})} =$$

$$\frac{\Delta n_g (c_{gp} - c_{gp'})}{\Delta n_f (q_{gp} - q_{gp'})} \leq R(A).$$

Thus if $h\hat{k}$ is cost-effective relative to hk

$$\frac{c_{h\hat{k}} - c_{hk}}{q_{h\hat{k}} - q_{hk}} \le R(A).$$

This last result establishes the necessity of the proposition's claim and the proof is complete.

Proposition 19. Let $h\hat{k}$ be added to the treatment for illness h and assume that $h\hat{k}$ does not strongly dominate and is not strongly dominated by another treatment hk. Then when $c_{h\hat{k}} < c_{hk}$ and $q_{h\hat{k}} < q_{hk}$, $h\hat{k}$ is cost-effective relative to hk if and only if

$$\frac{c_{hk} - c_{h\hat{k}}}{q_{hk} - q_{h\hat{k}}} \left[= \frac{c_{h\hat{k}} - c_{hk}}{q_{h\hat{k}} - q_{hk}} \right] \ge R(A).$$

In addition, treatments $h\hat{k}$ and hk are cost-effective relative to one another if and only if

$$\frac{c_{hk} - c_{h\hat{k}}}{q_{hk} - q_{h\hat{k}}} \left[= \frac{c_{h\hat{k}} - c_{hk}}{q_{h\hat{k}} - q_{hk}} \right] = R(A),$$

and total health benefits are the same whether patients are assigned to $h\hat{k}$ or hk.

Proof: There exists at least one pair of treatments gp and gp' such that $c_{gp} > c_{gp'}$, $q_{gp} > q_{gp'}$, $n_{gp'} > 0$, and

$$R(A) \ge \frac{c_{gp} - c_{gp'}}{q_{gp} - q_{gp'}}.$$

Again, for example, let gp = ij and gp' = ij'. Reassign Δn_h patients from hk to $h\hat{k}$ and Δn_g patients from gp' to gp so that $\Delta n_h(c_{h\hat{k}} - c_{hk}) - \Delta n_g(c_{gp} - c_{gp'}) = 0$. Suppose

$$\frac{c_{h\hat{k}} - c_{hk}}{q_{h\hat{k}} - q_{hk}} \ge R(A).$$

Hence it follows that

$$\frac{\Delta n_h(c_{h\hat{k}} - c_{hk})}{\Delta n_h(q_{h\hat{k}} - q_{hk})} \ge \frac{\Delta n_g(c_{gp} - c_{gp'})}{\Delta n_g(q_{gp} - q_{gp'})} = \frac{\Delta n_h(c_{h\hat{k}} - c_{hk})}{\Delta n_g(q_{gp} - q_{gp'})}$$

and $\Delta n_g(q_{gp} - q_{gp'}) \ge \Delta n_h(q_{h\hat{k}} - q_{hk})$. That is, with total cost fixed the reassignment increases or does not reduce total health benefits, and $h\hat{k}$ is therefore cost-effective relative to hk. Treatment $h\hat{k}$ is cost-effective relative to hk if

$$\frac{c_{h\hat{k}} - c_{hk}}{q_{h\hat{k}} - q_{hk}} > R(A).$$

If

$$\frac{c_{h\hat{k}} - c_{hk}}{q_{h\hat{k}} - q_{hk}} = R(A),$$

$h\hat{k}$ and hk are cost-effective relative to each other because $\Delta n_g(q_{gp} - q_{gp'}) = \Delta n_h(q_{h\hat{k}} - q_{hk})$ implies that with total cost fixed, total health benefits are not changed by switching patients back and forth from hk to $h\hat{k}$ and from $h\hat{k}$ to hk.

Next, suppose $h\hat{k}$ is cost-effective relative to hk. Then without changing total cost it must be possible to switch Δn_h patients from hk to $h\hat{k}$ and Δn_i patients from the less health-benefit productive treatment ij' for the cutoff-point illness i to the more health-benefit productive treatment ij so as to increase or not reduce total health benefits. In short, it must be true that with $\Delta n_h(c_{h\hat{k}} - c_{hk}) = \Delta n_i(c_{ij} - c_{ij'})$, $\Delta n_g(q_{ij} - q_{ij'}) \geq \Delta n_h(q_{h\hat{k}} - q_{hk})$. These two relations then imply

$$\frac{\Delta n_h(c_{h\hat{k}} - c_{hk})}{\Delta n_h(q_{h\hat{k}} - q_{hk})} \geq \frac{\Delta n_i(c_{ij} - c_{ij})}{\Delta n_i(q_{ij} - q_{ij'})} = R(A),$$

and if $h\hat{k}$ and hk are cost-effective relative to one another,

$$\frac{c_{h\hat{k}} - c_{hk}}{q_{h\hat{k}} - q_{hk}} = \frac{c_{ij} - c_{ij'}}{q_{ij} - q_{ij'}} = R(A).$$

Finally, if with total cost fixed, switching patients from $h\hat{k}$ to hk does not change total health benefits, it must be true that $\Delta n_h(c_{h\hat{k}} - c_{hk}) = \Delta n_i(c_{ij} - c_{ij'})$ and $\Delta n_g(q_{ij} - q_{ij'}) = \Delta n_h(q_{h\hat{k}} - q_{hk})$ for all gp and gp'. Hence it also follows that

$$\frac{c_{h\hat{k}} - c_{hk}}{q_{h\hat{k}} - q_{hk}} = \frac{c_{ij} - c_{ij'}}{q_{ij} - q_{ij'}} = R(A).$$

These last results complete the proof.

Notice especially that total treatment cost must be assumed constant during the switching procedure in order to prove $h\hat{k}$ is cost-effective relative to hk in Propositions 18 and 19. Obviously the two propositions are still valid if the switch of patients from hk to $h\hat{k}$ reduces total cost, but that is not so if total cost is allowed to increase—i.e., if $\Delta n_h(c_{h\hat{k}} - c_{hk}) > \Delta n_g(c_{gp} - c_{gp'})$ or $\Delta n_h(c_{h\hat{k}} - c_{hk}) > \Delta n_i(c_{ij} - c_{ij'})$. Therefore, if a health care agency is a myopic optimizer it cannot allow its total treatment cost to increase and still prove that $h\hat{k}$ is relatively cost-effective. Thus noninflationary treatment-choosing behavior is an integral feature of the MO model. Notice too that if $h\hat{k}$ is cost-effective relative to another treatment for h, switching patients to $h\hat{k}$ and reassigning patients among other treatments for other illnesses can cause some individuals to lose health benefits. As it is with the GM model, this result may seem damaging to the MO theory, but it is consistent with the principle that if $h\hat{k}$ is cost-effective in any sense, offering it to patients increases or does not reduce total health benefits. The community as a whole gains health wellbeing from the reassignment even though some individual patients may not.

The next proposition gives the first of the two MO rules for deciding the absolute cost-effectiveness of $h\hat{k}$. Proposition 21 gives the second rule.

Proposition 20. Let $h\hat{k}$ be a new nondominated treatment for h, where h may or may not be a cutoff-point illness. Add $h\hat{k}$ to the treatment set for h and remove all dominated treatments from the set. Then if $R_{h\hat{k}} \neq R(A)$, or if there is a treatment $h\hat{k}+1$ and $R_{h\hat{k}+1} \neq R(A)$, $h\hat{k}$ is absolutely cost-effective for illness h if and only if

$$(30) \qquad\qquad R_{h\hat{k}} = \max_m \{R_{hm} < R(A)\}$$

where each hm is in the new treatment set for h.

Proof: First suppose

181

$$R_{h\hat{k}} = \max_m \{R_{hm} < R(A)\}.$$

Hence by Proposition 5 the ordering of treatments in the new set causes $c_{h\hat{k}} > c_{hk}$, $q_{h\hat{k}} > q_{hk}$, and by Lemma 2,

$$R_{h\hat{k}} = \frac{c_{h\hat{k}} - c_{h\hat{k}-1}}{q_{h\hat{k}} - q_{h\hat{k}-1}} > \frac{c_{h\hat{k}} - c_{hk}}{q_{h\hat{k}} - q_{hk}}$$

for all $k \le \hat{k}$. Accordingly,

$$R(A) > R_{h\hat{k}} > \frac{c_{h\hat{k}} - c_{hk}}{q_{h\hat{k}} - q_{hk}}$$

for all hk such that $k \le \hat{k}$, and by Proposition 18 $h\hat{k}$ is cost-effective relative to each of these hk. Thus if there is no $h\hat{k} + 1$, $h\hat{k}$ is absolutely cost-effective for h. If there is a treatment $h\hat{k} + 1$, $R_{h\hat{k}}$ is the largest of the ICE ratios R_{hm} smaller than R(A), and inasmuch as $R_{h\hat{k}+1} \ne R(A)$. it must be that $R_{h\hat{k}+1} > R(A)$. Thus by the ordering of treatments in the new set, $c_{h\hat{k}} < c_{hk}$, $q_{h\hat{k}} < q_{hk}$, and by Lemma 2,

$$\frac{c_{hk} - c_{h\hat{k}}}{q_{hk} - q_{h\hat{k}}} > \frac{c_{h\hat{k}+1} - c_{h\hat{k}}}{q_{h\hat{k}+1} - q_{h\hat{k}}} = R_{h\hat{k}+1} > R(A)$$

for all $k > \hat{k}$. Therefore, by Proposition 19 $h\hat{k}$ is cost-effective relative to every hk such that $k > \hat{k}$, it is then cost-effective relative to every other treatment for h, and by that token it is absolutely cost-effective for h.

To prove necessity of the claim, suppose

$$R_{h\hat{k}} \ne \max_m \{R_{hm} < R(A)\}.$$

If

$$R_{h\hat{k}} < \max_m \{R_{hm} < R(A)\}$$

and $R_{h\hat{k}+1} \ne R(A)$, then

$$R_{h\hat{k}+1} = \frac{c_{h\hat{k}+1} - c_{h\hat{k}}}{q_{h\hat{k}+1} - q_{h\hat{k}}} < R(A)$$

as well. In that case $h\hat{k} + 1$ is cost-effective relative to $h\hat{k}$ by Proposition 18 (with $h\hat{k} + 1$ and $h\hat{k}$ replacing $h\hat{k}$ and $h\hat{k}$ replacing hk), and $h\hat{k}$ cannot be absolutely cost-effective for h. On the other hand, if

$$R_{h\hat{k}} > \max_{m} \{R_{hm} < R(A)\}$$

and $R_{h\hat{k}} \neq R(A)$,

$$R_{h\hat{k}} = \frac{c_{h\hat{k}} - c_{h\hat{k}-1}}{q_{h\hat{k}} - q_{h\hat{k}-1}} > R(A).$$

and by Proposition 19 $h\hat{k}$ -1 is then cost-effective relative to $h\hat{k}$ (with $h\hat{k}$ replacing hk and $h\hat{k}$ -1 replacing $h\hat{k}$). Hence again $h\hat{k}$ cannot be absolutely cost-effective for h. The argument has now shown that provided $R_{h\hat{k}}$, $R_{h\hat{k}+1} \neq R(A)$, treatment $h\hat{k}$ is absolutely cost-effective for h if (30) is true and not absolutely cost-effective otherwise. Thus the proof is complete.

Proposition 21. Let $h\hat{k}$ be a new nondominated treatment for h, where h may or may not be a cutoff-point illness. Add $h\hat{k}$ to the treatment set for h and remove all dominated treatments from the set. Then if $R_{h\hat{k}} =$ R(A) or $R_{h\hat{k}+1} = R(A)$, treatment $h\hat{k}$ can be declared absolutely cost-effective for h or not as the agency prefers, and with total cost fixed the total quantity of health benefits is the same whichever is the agency's choice.

Proof: Because the new treatment has no dominated members, Lemma 2 gives

$$\frac{c_{h\hat{k}} - c_{h\hat{k}-1}}{q_{h\hat{k}} - q_{h\hat{k}-1}} > \frac{c_{h\hat{k}} - c_{hk}}{q_{h\hat{k}} - q_{hk}} \text{ for all } k < \hat{k}$$

and

$$\frac{c_{hk} - c_{h\hat{k}}}{q_{hk} - q_{h\hat{k}}} > R_{h\hat{k}} = R(A) \text{ for all } k > \hat{k} .$$

Thus if

$$\frac{c_{h\hat{k}} - c_{h\hat{k}-1}}{q_{h\hat{k}} - q_{h\hat{k}-1}} = R(A),$$

$$R(A) > \frac{c_{h\hat{k}} - c_{hk}}{q_{h\hat{k}} - q_{hk}} \text{ for all } k < \hat{k}$$

and

$$R(A) < \frac{c_{hk} - c_{h\hat{k}}}{q_{hk} - q_{h\hat{k}}} \text{ for all } k > \hat{k} .$$

As a consequence, by Propositions 18 and 19 $h\hat{k}$ is cost-effective relative to every other treatment for h, and it is therefore absolutely cost-effective for h. However, $h\hat{k}-1$ is cost-effective relative to $h\hat{k}$ by Proposition 19, and therefore it is also cost-effective relative to every other treatment for h. Thus $h\hat{k}-1$ too is absolutely cost-effective for h. That is, either $h\hat{k}$ or $h\hat{k}-1$ can be declared absolutely cost-effective for h as the agency prefers.

Assume next that $R_{h\hat{k}+1}= R(A)$. Once more by Lemma 2,

$$R(A) = \frac{c_{h\hat{k}+1} - c_{h\hat{k}}}{q_{h\hat{k}+1} - q_{h\hat{k}}} > \frac{c_{h\hat{k}+1} - c_{hk}}{q_{h\hat{k}+1} - q_{hk}} \text{ for all } k < \hat{k}+1,$$

and

$$\frac{c_{hk} - c_{h\hat{k}+1}}{q_{hk} - q_{h\hat{k}+1}} > \frac{c_{h\hat{k}+1} - c_{h\hat{k}}}{q_{h\hat{k}+1} - q_{h\hat{k}}} = R(A) \text{ for all } k > \hat{k}+1.$$

Hence by Propositions 18 and 19 treatment $h\hat{k}+1$ is cost-effective relative to every other treatment for h and it is absolutely cost-effective for h. But by Proposition 19, $h\hat{k}$ is cost-effective relative to $h\hat{k}+1$ so that it is also absolutely cost-effective for h. Now either $h\hat{k}$ or $h\hat{k}+1$ can be declared absolutely cost-effective for h as the agency prefers.

Finally, if $R_{h\hat{k}} = R(A)$ or $R_{h\hat{k}+1}= R(A)$ with total cost fixed, by the proofs of Propositions 18 and 19 switching patients from hk to $h\hat{k}$ and back from $h\hat{k}$ to hk does not change total health benefits. Hence the agency neither gains nor loses health benefits by switching patients back and forth between $h\hat{k}$ and hk, and it is consequently indifferent as to which of the two treatments to offer to its patients. This result concludes the proof.

In Chapter 4 it was said that the $R_{h\hat{k}} = R(C)$ and $R_{h\hat{k}+1}= R(C)$ decision rules for a GM health care agency are vacuous when h = i because each equality implies that one of the treatments on with the ICE ratios $R_{h\hat{k}}$, $R_{h\hat{k}+1}$, and $R_{ik} = R(C)$ are defined is weakly dominated and the treatment will have been removed from the focal treatment set The same is also true for the myopic optimizer's $R_{h\hat{k}} = R(A)$ and $R_{h\hat{k}+1} = R(A)$ decision rules when h = i. The reasoning for the GM claim is given in Lemmas 7 and 8, and it obviously applies to the MO agency as well with ij' replacing ij-1 in the definition of the health care system's cutoff point.

7.3 Single-treatment Cost-effectiveness Analysis in the Myopic Optimizer Model: the Procedure and Examples

As in the GM model let $h\hat{k}$ be a new treatment for illness h, the focal illness. The steps in performing a single-treatment CEA for an MO health care agency are the same as those for a GM health care agency.

1. Determine or estimate the costs and health benefits of all treatments, including the new treatment $h\hat{k}$, for the focal illness h. Obtain the health care system's cutoff point R(A) or make it a parameter of the analysis.

2. Merge all nonstrictly strongly dominated treatments with the treatments that dominate them. If $c_{h\hat{k}} = c_{hk}$ and $q_{h\hat{k}} = q_{hk}$, merge $h\hat{k}$ and hk into a single treatment, and relabel the combined treatment $h\hat{k}$. Then remove all other dominated treatments, if there are any, from the new treatment set. If $h\hat{k}$ is dominated it is not absolutely cost-effective and the CEA terminates. If $h\hat{k}$ is not dominated, continue the CEA.

3. Order the remaining members of the treatment set so that costs and health benefits per patient increase strictly in the treatment index.

4. Compute the ICE ratios R_{h2}, R_{h3},..., $R_{h\hat{k}}$,..., R_{hK}. that are defined on adjacent treatments in the ordered set. Then the R_{hk} increase strictly in the treatment index k.

5. Determine whether

$$R_{h\hat{k}} = \frac{c_{h\hat{k}} - c_{h\hat{k}-1}}{q_{h\hat{k}} - q_{h\hat{k}-1}} = R(A)$$

or, if there is a treatment $h\hat{k} +1$, whether

$$R_{h\hat{k}+1} = \frac{c_{h\hat{k}+1} - c_{h\hat{k}}}{q_{h\hat{k}+1} - q_{h\hat{k}}} = R(A).$$

185

If $R_{h\hat{k}} = R(A)$ or $R_{h\hat{k}+1} = R(A)$, declare $h\hat{k}$ to be absolutely cost-effective for h or not as the agency prefers (Proposition 21). If $R_{h\hat{k}} \neq R(A)$ and $R_{h\hat{k}+1} \neq R(A)$, go to Step 6.

   6. Apply the maximum ICE-ratio decision rule of Proposition 20: conclude that $h\hat{k}$ is absolutely cost-effective for h if and only if

$$R_{h\hat{k}} = \max_{m} \{R_{hm} < R(A) \}.$$

If $R(A)$ cannot be reliably obtained or estimated, conclude that $h\hat{k}$ is absolutely cost-effective for h if and only if $R_{h\hat{k}} < R(A) < R_{h\hat{k}+1}$ when there is a treatment $h\hat{k} + 1$ and otherwise if and only if $R(A) > R_{h\hat{k}}$.

   Four numerical examples of single-treatment MO CEA are now given to illustrate the use of the decision rules They are not intended to be realistic. To provide comparability with the examples of single-treatment GM CEAs, the population sizes, the set of all treatments for all illnesses, and treatment costs and health benefit products are the same as those of Chapter 6. Table 7.1 is identical to Table 6.1. In addition, the examples assume the same total treatment cost of $10.5 million used in the first of the GM examples given in Chapter 6.

   Suppose the MO agency's initial global patient assignment is as it is shown in Table 7.2. Thus at the total cost of $10.5 million the total quantity of health benefits produced by the MO agency is 2,131.96 units and its cutoff point is $34,000 per unit of health benefits. That is, illness 1 is the cutoff-point illness and

$$R_{13} = \frac{c_{13} - c_{12}}{q_{13} - q_{12}} = \$34,000 \text{ per unit of health benefits}$$

is the largest observed ICE ratio defined on any pair of treatments such that positive numbers of patients are assigned to each member of the pair. By way of contrast, the GM agency having the same treatment cost and health benefits data produces 2,217.6 units of health benefits at the total cost $10.5 million, and its cutoff point is $25,000 per unit of health benefits.

Table 7.1
Treatment Costs, Health Benefits, Incremental Cost-Effectiveness Ratios, and Patient Populations in an Illustrative Health Care System

Treatment	Cost per Treatment in $ (c_{hk})	Health Benefits per Treatment (q_{hk})	ICE Ratio ($ per Benefit)	Patient Population
11	0	0	--	200
12	2,300	0.4	6,000	
13	7,500	0.55	34,000	
21	0	0	--	300
22	8,000	1.0	8,000	
23	12,000	1.16	25,000	
31	0	0	--	300
32	250	0.1	2,500	
33	1,000	0.25	5,000	
34	2,200	0.3	24,000	
41	0	0	--	200
42	1,500	0.4	3,750	
43	5,000	0.75	10,000	
44	18,000	1.25	26,000	
51	0	0	--	300
52	600	3.0	200	
53	2,450	3.5	3,700	
54	5,200	4.0	5,500	
55	6,600	4.2	7,000	
56	10,000	4.4	17,000	

Table 7.2
Treatments to Which Positive numbers of Patients Are Initially Assigned by a Myopic Optimizing Health Care Agency

Illness	Treatment	ICE Ratio in $ Per Unit	Number of Patients Assigned to Treatment	Total Cost of Treatment in Millions of $	Total Health Benefits Produced by Treatment
1	12	6,000	243	0.5832	97.2
	13	**34,000**	257	1.9275	131.25
2	22	8,000	144	1.152	144
	23	25,000	256	3.072	296.96
3	31	--	12	0	0
	32	2,500	82	0.0205	8.2
	33	5,000	206	0.206	51.5
4	42	3,750	99	0.1485	29.6
	43	10,000	53	0.265	29.75
	44	26,000	48	0.864	60
5	52	200	20	0.012	60
	53	3,700	10	0.0245	35
	54	5,500	14	0.0728	56
	55	7,000	120	0.792	504
	56	17,000	136	1.36	598.4
Total, All Treatments			1,700	10.5	2,131.96

C = $10.5 million. Cutoff point in boldface.

Example 1. Suppose a new treatment 3a costing $1,600 and producing 0.29 units of health benefits becomes available for illness 3. Illness 3 is the focal illness and the new treatment set for illness 3 is shown in Table 7.3. None of the five treatments in the set is dominated. By inspection of Table 7.3, $R_{3a} = 15,000 \neq R_{34}$ (= $R_{h\hat{k}}$), and the appropriate rule for deciding the absolute cost-effectiveness is therefore the maximum ICE-ratio rule of step 6. Also by inspection of Table 7.3,

$$R_{3a} = \max_m \{R_{3m} < 34,000)\}$$

so that treatment 3a is absolutely cost-effective for illness 3 by the maximum ICE-ratio rule.

The MO analyst would not need to know anything more than the decision rule's conclusion, but to see that the conclusion is correct, consider first the reassignments of patients to treatment 3a from treatments 31, 32, and 33. Treatment 3a is more costly than each of these three treatments, so to offset the increase in total cost resulting in each of the reassignments, patients having illness 1 can be switched from the more expensive treatment 13 (for the cutoff-point illness 1) to the less

Table 7.3
Example 1. Treatment Costs, Health Benefits, and Incremental Cost-Effectiveness Ratios for the New Treatment Set for Illness 3

Treatment	Cost per Treatment in $ (c_{3m})	Health Benefits per Treatment (q_{3m})	ICE Ratio in $ Per Unit of Health Benefits
31	0	0	--
32	250	0.1	2,500
33	1,000	0.25	5,000
3a	1,600	0.29	15,000
34	2,200	0.3	60,000

Table 7.4
Example 1. Per-Patient Net Change in Health Benefits When One Patient Is Reassigned from Treatments 31, 32, and 33 to 3a and Other Patients are Reassigned from Treatment 13 to Treatment 12 with Total Cost Constant

Re-assignment to 3a	Cost Increase ($)	Health Bene-fits Increase (units)	Number of Patients Switched from 13 to 12 to Maintain Constant Total Cost [(Column 2 ÷ (5,100)]*	Loss of Health Benefits Due to Switching Patients From 13 to 12 (Column 4 x 0.15)*	Net Change in Health Benefits (Column 3 – Column 5)
31 → 3a	1,600	0.29	0.314	0.047	0.233
32 → 3a	1,350	0.19	0.265	0.030	0.150
33 → 3a	600	0.04	0.118	0.018	0.022

*Reassigning one patient from treatment 13 to treatment 12 reduces total cost by $5,100 and reduces total health benefits by 0.15 units.

expensive treatment 12. The effects of the reassignments are displayed in in Table 7.4. As shown in column 6 of the Table, each of the three reassignments increases total health benefits with total cost constant, and these results are sufficient to prove that 3a is cost-effective relative to each of the treatments 31, 32, and 33.

Now (hypothetically) consider reassigning patients from treatment 34 to treatment 3a. The switch causes a loss of health benefits, but to compensate for the loss patients having illness 1 can be switched from treatment 12 to treatment 13. (Given the definition of the cutoff point, it is always provable that patients can be switched from the less health-benefit productive of the two treatments that define the cutoff point to the more health-benefit productive treatment.) When one patient is switched from 34 to 3a there occurs a reduction of $600 in total cost and a loss of 0.01 units of health benefits. To maintain the constancy of total cost, 0.5 (=

$600÷$1,200) patients can be switched from treatment 12 to treatment 13, and the gain in total health benefits is 0.025 (= 0.5x0.05) units. Hence the net change in total health benefits is 0.15 (= 0.025 – 0.01) units per patient and this result demonstrates that 3a is cost-effective relative to 34.

In sum, these numerical calculations indicate that 3a is cost-effective relative to every other treatment for focal illness 3 and therefore that it is absolutely cost-effective for the illness.

If the analyst does not know and cannot reliably estimate the cutoff point, her report at the completion of the CEA should be the same as that if the health care agency were GM. She should inform the agency that treatment 3a

- is not absolutely cost-effective if R(A) < $15,000 per unit of health benefits;
- can be declared absolutely cost-effective or not if R(A) = $15,000 per unit of health benefits;
- Is absolutely cost-effective if $15,000 < R(A) < $60,000 per unit of health benefits;
- can be declared absolutely cost-effective or not if R(A) = $60,000 per unit of health benefits;
- is not absolutely cost-effective if R(A) > $60,000 per unit of health benefits.

Example 2. Let the initial treatment set be the same as in Example 1 (Table 7.1), and assume the initial global assignment is the same as well (Table 7.2). Then as in Example 1 the health care system's cutoff point is $34,000 per unit of health benefits. But assume the focal illness is illness 1 and that a new treatment for the illness labeled 1a becomes available to the agency. The cost of 1a is $5,300 per patient and the treatment produces 0.52 units of health benefits per patient. The members of the new treatment set are shown in Table 7.5. None of the members of the set is dominated, and there are no ICE ratios equal to the cutoff point. Then as in Example 1 the appropriate decision rule for

Table 7.5
Example 2. Treatment Costs, Health Benefits, and Incremental Cost-Effectiveness Ratios for the New Treatment Set for Illness 1

Treatment	Cost per Treatment in $ (c_{1m})	Health Benefits per Treatment (q_{1m})	ICE Ratio in $ Per Unit of Health Benefits
11	0	0	--
12	2,300	0.4	6,000
1a	5,300	0.52	25,000
13	7,500	0.55	70,000

assessing the absolute cost-effectiveness of 1a is the maximum ICE-ratio rule 6. Thus the only difference between Examples 1 and 2 is that the focal illness in Example 2 is the cutoff-point illness and the focal illness in Example 1 is not.

By inspection of Table 7.5 it is evident that R_{1a} is the largest of the ICE ratios in the new treatment set that is smaller than the cutoff point $34,000 per unit of health benefits. Therefore, by the maximum ICE-ratio decision rule 6, treatment 1a is absolutely cost-effective for illness 1. To verify the correctness of the decision, consider the consequences of switching patients to 1a from each of the other treatments for illness 1, 11, 12, and 13. These are summarized in Table 7.6. For example, switching a single patient from 12 to 1a increases total cost by $3,000 (= $5,300 - $2,300) and increases total health benefits by 0.12 units. To compensate for the increase in total cost, 1.059 (= $3,000÷$5,100) patients must be switched from treatment 13 to treatment 12. This compensating reassignment of patients reduces total health benefits by 0.088 [= 1.059x(0.55 – 0.4)] units, but the net change in total health

Table 7.6
Example 2. Per-Patient Net Change in Health Benefits When One Patient Is Reassigned from Treatments 11, 12, and 13 to 1a and Other Patients are Reassigned from Treatment 13 to Treatment 12 and from Treatment 13 to Treatment 12 with Total Cost Constant

Reas-sign-ment	Change in Total Cost ($)	Change in Total Health Benefits (units)	Patients Switched from 12 to 13 to Maintain Constant Total Cost (Col. 2 ÷ 5,100)*	Patients Switched from 13 to 12 to Maintain Constant Total Cost [(Col. 2) ÷ (5,100)]	Loss of Health Benefits from Compen-sating Reas-signment (Col. 4 or 5 x 0.15)*	Net Change in Total Health Benefits (Col. 3 – Col. 6)
11→1a	5,300	0.52	1.059	--	0.158	0.362
12→1a	3,000	0.12	0.588	--	0.088	0.032
13→1a	-2,100	-0.03	--	0.312	-0.062	0.032

*Reassigning one patient from treatment 13 to treatment 12 reduces total cost by $5,100 and reduces total health benefits by 0.15 units.

benefits is 0.32 (= 0.12 – 0.088) units, and as a result treatment 1a is cost-effective relative to treatment 12. When one patient is switched from treatment 13 to treatment 1a total cost is reduced by $2,100 and total health benefits are reduced by 0.03 units. If total cost is held constant, 0.312 (= 2,100 ÷ 5,100) patients must be switched from treatment 12 to treatment 13, and this reassignment causes a gain of 0.062 units of health benefits. Accordingly, switching each patient from treatment 13 to treatment 1a and compensating the reduction in costs by switching 0.312 patients from treatment 12 to treatment 13 yields a net gain of 0.032 (= 0.062 – 0.03) units of health benefits. All three reassignments of patients to 1a from other treatments for illness 1 give positive gains in total health benefits, and as a consequence the calculations confirm the correctness of the cost-effectiveness decision rule 6.

Example 3. Again suppose the initial treatment set and global patient assignment are the same as in Example 1. As before the health care system's cutoff point is $34,000 per unit of health benefits, but suppose the focal illness is illness 2 and a new treatment 2a becomes available for the illness. Assume the cost of 2a is $15,000 per patient and that the treatment yields 1.21 units of health benefits per patient. The new treatment set for illness 2 is shown in Table 7.7. None of the treatments is dominated and it is evident from the table that R_{2a} (= $R_{h\hat{k}}$) is not equal to the health care system's cutoff point. Thus as in the first two examples the appropriate decision rule is the maximum ICE-ratio rule 6. Then R_{2a} = 50,000 > max $\{R_{2m}$ < 34,000\}, and it follows from the rule that 2a is not absolutely cost-effective for illness 2. Hence the agency should not provide or sanction treatment 2a for its patients having illness 2.

Table 7.7
Example 3. Treatment Costs, Health Benefits, and Incremental Cost-Effectiveness Ratios for the New Treatment Set for Illness 2

Treatment	Cost per Treatment in $ (c_{1m})	Health Benefits per Treatment (q_{1m})	ICE Ratio in $ Per Unit of Health Benefits
21	0	0	--
22	8,000	1	8,000
23	12,000	1.16	25,000
2a	15,000	1.21	50,000

To verify the conclusion that 2a is not absolutely cost-effective for illness 2, it is sufficient to show that 2a is not cost-effective relative to at least one other treatment for illness 2. Suppose then that patients have been assigned to 2a and that one or more of them are reassigned to treatment 23. For each such patient so reassigned total cost is reduced by $3,000 and total health benefits are reduced by 0.05 units. To offset the reduction in total cost assume patients are switched from treatment 12

194

to treatment 13, the two treatments that define the health care system's cutoff point. Each patient switched from 12 to 13 increases total cost by $5,200 and increases total health benefits by 0.15 units. Hence for each $3,000 reduction in total cost as a patient is switched from 2a to 23, 0.588 (= $3,000÷$5,200) patients must be switched from treatment 12 to treatment 13. The latter reassignment increases total health benefits by 0.0882 (= 0.15x0.588) units, and therefore the net change in total health benefits produced by cost-constrained reassignment of patients from treatment 2a to treatment 23 and from treatment 12 to treatment 13 is 0.0882 − 0.05 = 0.0382 units. Since the reassignment increases total net benefits without increasing total cost, 23 is cost-effective relative to 2a and 2a therefore cannot be absolutely cost-effective for illness 2.

Example 4. Once more let the initial treatment set and global patient assignment be the same as in Example 1. The health care system's cutoff point is still $34,000 per unit of health benefits. As in Example 3 assume the focal illness is illness 2 and a new treatment 2a becomes available for the illness. But now assume the cost of 2a is $13,360 per patient and that 2a produces 1.2 units of health benefits per patient. The new treatment set for 2a is shown in Table 7.8, and R_{2a} is $34,000 per unit of health benefits. Since R_{2a} (= $R_{h\hat{k}}$) equals the health

Table 7.8
Example 4. Treatment Costs, Health Benefits, and Incremental Cost-Effectiveness Ratios for the New Treatment Set for Illness 2

Treatment	Cost per Treatment in $ (c_{1m})	Health Benefits per Treatment (q_{1m})	ICE Ratio in $ Per Unit of Health Benefits
21	0	0	--
22	8,000	1	8,000
23	12,000	1.16	25,000
2a	13,360	1.2	34,000

care system's cutoff point, the applicable rule for deciding the absolute cost-effectiveness of 2a is the $R_{h\hat{k}} = R(A)$ decision rule 5 in the CEA procedure, and by that rule 2a can be declared absolutely cost-effective or not for illness 2 as the agency prefers. To establish the correctness of the rule for the example it must be demonstrated that 2a is cost-effective relative to each of the other treatments for illness 2, and that the second most expensive, most health-benefit productive treatment for the illness, 23 (= $R_{h\hat{k}-1}$) is also cost-effective relative to 2a. That 2a is cost-effective relative to treatments 21, 22, and 23 is shown in Table 7.9. In the table it is assumed that patients are switched from treatment 13 to treatment 12 to offset the cost increases caused be reassigning one patient to 2a from each of the other treatments for illness 2 and it is therefore absolutely cost-effective for the illness. Comparable calculations for reassignments of patients from 21, 22, and 2a to treatment 23 are given in Table 7.10. In the rightmost column of the table it is shown that with total cost fixed, switching patients from treatments 21, 22, and 2a to treatment 23 also increases or does not reduce health benefits. Hence 23 is provably cost-effective relative to each of these treatments and as a consequence it too is absolutely cost-effective for illness 2. With total cost fixed the net change in total health benefits that can be attained by switching patients from 2a to 23 is zero—just as is the net change attainable from switching patients from 23 to 2a.

The computations shown in Tables 7.9 and 7.10 corroborate the finding given by the $R_{h\hat{k}} = R(A)$ decision rule. Treatments 2a and 23 are both absolutely cost-effective for illness 2, and as a result the MO agency should be indifferent as to which of the treatments for illness 2 it should provide to or insure for its patients. In the rightmost column of Table 10 it can be seen that the reassignments from 21 and 22 to 2a bring about increases in total health benefits, but the reassignment from 23 to 2a causes no change. Thus the numbers in the table prove that, with total costs fixed, global assignments exist in which 2a is provided to

Table 7.9
Example 4. Per-Patient Net Change in Health Benefits When One Patient Is Reassigned from Treatments 21, 22, and 23 to 2a and Other Patients are Reassigned from Treatment 13 to Treatment 12 with Total Cost Constant

Reas-sign-ment	Change in Total Cost ($)	Change in Total Health Benefits (units)	Patients Switched from 12 to 13 to Maintain Constant Total Cost (Col. 2 ÷ 5,100)*	Patients Switched from 13 to 12 to Maintain Constant Total Cost [(Col. 2) ÷ (5,100)]	Loss of Health Benefits from Compen-sating Reas-signment (Col. 4 or 5 x 0.15)*	Net Change in Total Health Benefits (Col. 3 – Col. 6)
21→2a	13,360	1.2	2.260	0.393	0.158	0.807
22→2a	5,360	0.2	1.051	0.158	0.088	0.042
23→2a	1,360	0.04	0.267	--	0.04	0

*Switching one patient from treatment 13 to treatment 12 reduces total cost by $5,100 and reduces total health benefits by 0.15 units.

or sanctioned for patients, and these assignments yield quantities of health benefits that are at least as large as the quantities attainable by not providing or sanctioning 2a for patients. Accordingly, treatment 2a is cost-effective relative to each of the other two treatments the agency provides to or sanctions for its patients. When total cost is constant, patients initially assigned to treatment 22 (and to treatment 21 if n_{21} had been positive) can be reassigned to either 2a and 23 and the same quantity of health benefits can be obtained.

To make the same point in a slightly different way, compare the figures in the rightmost columns of Tables 7.9 and 7.10. The figures in this column of Table 7.9 show the gains in total health benefits obtained when one patient is switched to treatment 2a from treatments 21, 22, and 23 with total cost fixed.   The figures in the rightmost column of Table 7.10

Table 7.10
Example 4. Per-Patient Net Change in Health Benefits When One Patient Is Reassigned from Treatments 11, 12, and 13 to 2a and Other Patients are Reassigned from Treatment 13 to Treatment 12 and from Treatment 13 to Treatment 12 with Total Cost Constant

Reas-sign-ment	Change in Total Cost ($)	Change in Total Health Benefits (units)	Patients Switched from 12 to 13 to Maintain Constant Total Cost (Col. 2 ÷ 5,100)*	Patients Switched from 13 to 12 to Maintain Constant Total Cost [(Col. 2) ÷ (5,100)]	Loss of Health Benefits from Compen-sating Reas-signmen t (Col. 4 or 5 x 0.15)*	Net Change in Total Health Benefits (Col. 3 – Col. 6)
21→23	12,000	1.16	2.353	--	0.353	0.807
22→23	4,000	0.16	0.784	--	0.118	0.042
2a→23	- 1,360	- 0.04	--	0.267	-0.04	0

*Switching one patient from treatment 13 to treatment 12 reduces total cost by $5,100 and reduces total health benefits by 0.15 units.

show the gains in total health benefits obtained when one patient is switched to treatment 23 from treatments 21, 22, and 2a, also with total cost fixed. Observe that switching one patient from 21 to 2a yields exactly the same cost-constrained increase in total health benefits as switching the same patient from 21 to 23, and that switching one patient from 22 to 2a yields exactly the same cost-constrained increase in total health benefits as switching the same patient from 22 to 23. Finally, there are no cost-constrained gains in total health benefits to be made by switching a patient from 23 to 2a or back again from 2a to 23. Hence there are no advantages or disadvantages in reassigning patients having illness h from the other treatments for the illness to 2a rather than 23 or to 23 rather than 2a. These results also illustrate the fact that 2a and 23 are both absolutely cost-effective for illness h, and that it is myopically optimal to assign patients having h to 2a, 23, or to some combination of the two treatments.

The foregoing examples show—and it is important to emphasize—that the MO decision rules indicate only that there exists or does not exist a myopic reassignment of patients that makes a new treatment absolutely cost-effective. Nothing in the rules informs the health care agency how to reassign patients when $\hat{hk}$ is judged absolutely cost-effective. As it is in the GM model, the MO agency must itself find the new assignment, perhaps along the lines of the searches suggested by the examples here. The cost-effectiveness analyst is responsible only proving that the reassignment can be made and not what it is.

7.4 The Equivalence of the Myopic Optimizer and GM Decision Rules

A comparison of the 6-step MO and GM procedures for single-treatment CEA given in Sections 7.3 and 6.1 shows that the MO and GM decision rules are identical except possibly in the unlikely event that C equals the GM agency's budget point C^t. Budget points have no part in the MO decision rules. In both procedures the dominated members of the new treatment set for h are removed, the nondominated treatments are ordered in exactly the same way, and the decision rules of steps 5 and 6 are identical as well. Thus the same CEA can be applied to test the absolute cost-effectiveness of a new treatment when the health care agency is either a myopic optimizer or a global maximizer, and the six-step procedure can be defended both logically and ethically whichever is the type of the agency. Indeed, because the assumptions on the optimizing behavior of the MO agency are less stringent than those on the optimizing behavior of the GM agency, it does no harm to posit always that the agency is MO. If the surmise is incorrect, the CEA's judgement of the absolute cost-effectiveness of $h\hat{k}$ for the GM agency is still valid.

When all treatment costs and health benefits are the same, myopic optimizer and global maximizer CEAs will give the same conclusion for the absolute cost-effectiveness of $h\hat{k}$ if two conditions are satisfied:

(i) R(A) = R(C) and

(ii) for the GM agency, $C \neq C^t$ for all t.

It is unnecessary, however, to know that the two conditions are or are not satisfied. The CEA's conclusion hinges only on the result that $h\hat{k}$ is or is not dominated and the value of the health care system's cutoff point. That fact that $h\hat{k}$ is or is not dominated is the same for both types of agencies, and the health care system's cutoff point is either a fixed piece of information for the analyst whatever is the agency's optimizing behavior or else a parameter of the analysis. In either event, the analyst need not specify the health care agency's behavior in order to perform a single-treatment CEA and justify its result.

The methods of single-treatment CEA are founded here on the premise that the health care agency is either GM or MO, and they might be challenged on grounds that a typical agency is not necessarily either GM nor MO. But the challenge is irrelevant. The MO model makes no suppositions about the agency's goal behavior prior to the application of the six-step single-treatment CEA procedure. The agency may have exhibited any kind of goal behavior or it may not have pursued a consistent or rational institutional goal. Whatever its past administrative conduct may have been, the agency becomes a myopic optimizer simply by adopting the MO procedure and the MO decision rules. Hence, for example, a state Medicaid program or a national or provincial health service need not be radically restructured in order to make it a more efficient producer of health wellbeing. All that it is required is that the agency begin acting as a myopic optimizer. The agency then becomes efficient only incrementally, and it will not produce as high a level of its community's health wellbeing as it would if it were a global maximizer.

Nevertheless, it will produce a higher level of health wellbeing than an agency lacking or unable to implement the objective of producing more than fewer health benefits for its community.

7.5   On the Existence of the Myopic Optimizer's Cutoff Point

A key premise of the MO agency model is that there exists an observable cutoff point R(A) and thus that there must exist at least one illness g and two treatments gp and gp' for the illness such that n_{gp} and $n_{gp'}$ are both initially positive. The premise is standard in the traditional procedures of single-treatment CEA and it is likely to be satisfied in most empirical situations. But there are no theoretical reasons for believing it must be so. If the health care agency is GM and $C = C^t$, all patients having each illness are initially assigned to exactly one treatment for each illness. And even if the agency is not GM, it may can always choose to assign patients to only one treatment for each of the illnesses it cares for.

To prove relative cost-effectiveness in Proposition 19 it must be possible to switch patients having illness h between $h\hat{k}$ and hk and to switch patients having another illness g between gp and gp' so as to preserve the constancy of total treatment cost. Then $h\hat{k}$ is or is not cost-effective relative to hk depending on how the myopic reassignment changes total health benefits. The switch of patients between $h\hat{k}$ and hk can be hypothetical but the switch between gp and gp' cannot because the change in health benefits generally varies with the designations of g, gp, and gp', and the conclusion that $h\hat{k}$ is or is not relatively cost-effective therefore varies as well. Suppose the agency initially assigns patients to only one treatment for every illness. It is not impossible to define a cutoff point in that case, but to do so the analyst must select a candidate illness g and either gp or gp' since patients are assigned to only one of the two treatments. There are no obvious theoretical lines of argument for doing either of these things, and if two different analysts were to undertake them there can be no assurances that they would choose the same illness g or, if they did, they would also choose the same pair of treatments ij and ij'. Hence there can be no assurance that they would reach the same conclusion about the relative and absolute cost-effectiveness of $h\hat{k}$. In short, if the agency does not initially assign patients to two or more treatments for at least one illness, there exist no definitive rules for assessing relative and absolute cost-effectiveness.

That it cannot be proved that $h\hat{k}$ is or is not (relative and) absolutely cost-effective when the agency assigns patients to only one treatment for each illness is an obvious shortcoming of the MO model. If the analyst discovers that the agency for which the CEA is performed assigns patients to only one treatment for each illness, she should report simply and correctly that an MO CEA of the new treatment $h\hat{k}$ is not feasible. The agency and analyst can, of course, resort to some other rules such as those using arbitrary or willingness-to-pay cutoff points for deciding the absolute cost-effectiveness of $h\hat{k}$, but then the welfare implications of the decision are readily questionable.

8 Single-Treatment Cost-Effectiveness Analysis and The Deterministic Theory of Net Benefits

8.1 Introduction

The theory of net benefits is not a theory of health care agency behavior but instead a theory—if that is an appropriate word for it—of a special and particularly useful decision variable for single-treatment CEA. What might be called the classical decision variable for single-treatment CEA is an ICE ratio, and until roughly two decades ago it was regarded as perfectly acceptable for empirical analyses. CEAs were performed deterministically—that is, with single-valued estimates of treatment costs and health benefits, and the decision that a new treatment was or was not cost-effective was made by comparing a single-valued ICE ratio with an assumed cutoff point.

However, beginning in the 1980s and 1990s sample data on treatment costs and health benefits began to be available or could be generated by methods such as Monte Carlo simulation, and it became evident to many analysts that single-treatment CEAs could be conducted probabilistically. But when there are multiple values of costs and health benefits in a natural or constructed sample of data on treatments, there are also multiple values of $R_{h\hat{k}}$ and the other ICE ratios R_{hk}. Thus, depending on the sample values of ICE ratios, decision rules such as the maximum ICE-ratio rule (29) could imply that $h\hat{k}$ is or is not relatively or absolutely cost-effective. In short, as soon as sample data on treatment costs and health benefits are used in single treatment CEAs, costs, health benefits, ICE ratios, and the yes-no or 0-1 conclusions of the analyses all become random variables. Hence to perform single-treatment CEAs using sample data some kind of statistical methodology had to be adopted or created to perform the analyses. Insofar as ICE ratios are the principle decision variables of single-treatment CEAs this requirement immediately raised a problem, for except under unusual and hard-to-imagine conditions it cannot be assumed that an ICE ratio has a tractable sample distribution, one, for example, that yields meaningful inferences about the ratio's mean and variance. The issue is discussed in Chapter 9 and it is remarked here only because this statistical problem with ICE ratios gave rise to the theory of net benefits.

It is not altogether clear who originated the idea of net benefits, but the first explicit discussion of the concept is by Stinnett and Mullahy [1998]. Stinnet and Mullahy defined a new decision variable for single-treatment CEAs, and called it the "net health benefit" the treatment produces. Subsequently a slightly more aesthetically attractive variation of the net health benefit variable was created by researchers and dubbed the treatment's "net monetary benefit".

Definitions. Let R denote the health care system's cutoff point in whatever way it is specified. Then the net health benefit of treatment hk is
$$NHB_{hk} = q_{hk} - c_{hk}/R,$$
and the net monetary benefit of treatment hk is
$$NMB_{hk} = Rq_{hk} - c_{hk}.$$
Since $NMB_{hk} = NHB_{hk}xR$, the two variables are interchangeable, and rather than dealing with them separately or distinguishing between net monetary benefits and net health benefits, *hereafter net benefits will be defined as net monetary benefits and abbreviated to*
$$B_{hk} = Rq_{hk} - c_{hk}.$$
The incremental net benefit of treatment hk relative to treatment hk' is
$$B_{hkk'} = B_{hk} - B_{hk'} = R(q_{hk} - q_{hk'}) - (c_{hk} - c_{hk'}).$$

Unlike an ICE ratio which can be understood either as a marginal cost of health benefits or as a price of health benefits, neither the net benefit of a treatment nor the incremental net benefit of two treatments has a sensible economic interpretation. But because B_{hk} and $B_{hkk'}$ are linear combinations of treatment cost and health benefits, taken as random variables they can ordinarily be assumed to have manageable sampling distributions. That is, it can reasonably be assumed that treatment costs and health benefits are or are approximately normally distributed, especially if they are taken as large-sample means. Hence with R fixed it follows that B_{hk} and $B_{hkk'}$ are or are approximately normally distributed as well, and ordinary normal-based statistical tests on the parameters of the distributions of B_{hk} and $B_{hkk'}$ become feasible. The question then is how to make use of this convenient statistical property by showing that logical tests of relative and absolute cost-effectiveness can be conducted with the use of the net benefits variables. The next section of this chapter is devoted to that end.

8.2 The Deterministic Theory of Net Benefits

Although the net benefits variable was first defined so as to make probabilistic judgments of cost-effectiveness a simple matter, the logic of the net benefits single-treatment decision rules is best explained by assuming the rules are deterministic and that assumption will be maintained throughout this chapter. Because all decision rules are meant to enable their users to achieve a worthwhile objective, it is also supposed that a health care agency adopts the net benefits rules in order to allow it to increase or maximize the health wellbeing of its community. Two health care agency models have been proposed in this book, the global maximizer and myopic optimizer models. It is possible that other health welfare models can be used to rationalize the net benefits decision rules, but here and because it is generally the less restrictive of the GM and MO models, *to begin with it will be assumed that a health care agency employing the net benefits rules is a myopic optimizer.*

It has become commonplace in the CEA literature to present and discuss the net benefits theory with the cutoff point R specified as the health care agency's or the agency's community's willingness to pay an additional unit of health benefits. That the concepts of net benefits and willingness to pay have evolved together is, however, merely a historical accident, and the two are in no way linked either logically or empirically.

Under certain circumstances (i.e., when is observed) it is possible to understand R as a willingness to pay, but as was argued in Chapter 5 the rationality of the principle of willingness to pay is at best debatable. For that reason it will not be assumed that R is a willingness to pay. It will be assumed first that $R = R(A)$, an MO agency's cutoff point. In the next section it is shown that a GM health care agency can also use the net benefits decision rules, and therefore R can be taken either as an MO agency's cutoff point or $R(C)$, the cutoff point of a global maximizer.

It will be recalled that in the procedure of a single-treatment MO CEA all nonstrictly strongly dominated members of the new treatment set for h—i.e., including the new treatment $h\hat{k}$—are merged with the treatments that dominate them. Thus all remaining strongly dominated treatments in the set are strictly strongly dominated. Then $h\hat{k}$ either strongly dominates another treatment hk or it does not. If it does, it is cost-effective relative to hk. If $h\hat{k}$ does not strongly dominate hk, either $c_{h\hat{k}} >$ c_{hk}, $q_{h\hat{k}} > q_{hk}$ or $c_{h\hat{k}} < c_{hk}$, $q_{h\hat{k}} < q_{hk}$ and by Propositions 18 and 19 $h\hat{k}$ is cost-effective relative to hk if and only if

(31) $$\frac{c_{h\hat{k}} - c_{hk}}{q_{h\hat{k}} - q_{hk}} \leq R(A) \text{ when } c_{h\hat{k}} > c_{hk}, q_{h\hat{k}} > q_{hk},$$

and

(32) $$\frac{c_{hk} - c_{h\hat{k}}}{q_{hk} - q_{h\hat{k}}} \geq R(A) \text{ when } c_{h\hat{k}} < c_{hk}, q_{h\hat{k}} < q_{hk}.$$

Proposition 22 that follows gives necessary and sufficient conditions on the net benefits of $h\hat{k}$ and hk for $h\hat{k}$ to be cost-effective relative to hk. Proposition 23 gives necessary and sufficient conditions on the net benefits $h\hat{k}$ and all other treatments for h for $h\hat{k}$ to be absolutely cost-effective for h.

Proposition 22. Let $h\hat{k}$ and hk be any two treatments for the same illness h. Then $h\hat{k}$ is cost-effective relative to hk if and only if $B_{h\hat{k}} \geq B_{hk}$. If $B_{h\hat{k}} = B_{hk}$, $h\hat{k}$ and hk are each cost-effective relative to the other.

Proof: Treatment $h\hat{k}$ strictly strongly dominates hk or it does not. If it does, $h\hat{k}$ is cost-effective relative to hk, $c_{h\hat{k}} \leq c_{hk}$, $q_{h\hat{k}} \geq q_{hk}$ where at least one of the inequalities is strict, and $B_{h\hat{k}} - B_{hk} = R(q_{h\hat{k}} - q_{hk}) + (c_{h\hat{k}} - c_{hk}) > 0$.

Now suppose $h\hat{k}$ does not strongly dominate hk. Since neither $h\hat{k}$ nor hk dominates the other treatment, either $c_{h\hat{k}} > c_{hk}$ and $q_{h\hat{k}} > q_{hk}$ or $c_{h\hat{k}} < c_{hk}$ and $q_{h\hat{k}} < q_{hk}$. So consider

$$(33) \qquad B_{h\hat{k}} - B_{hk} = (q_{h\hat{k}} - q_{hk})\left[R - \frac{c_{h\hat{k}} - c_{hk}}{q_{h\hat{k}} - q_{hk}}\right] \text{ if } c_{h\hat{k}} > c_{hk}, q_{h\hat{k}} > q_{hk},$$

and

$$(34) \qquad B_{hk} - B_{h\hat{k}} = (q_{hk} - q_{h\hat{k}})\left[R - \frac{c_{hk} - c_{h\hat{k}}}{q_{hk} - q_{h\hat{k}}}\right] \text{ if } c_{h\hat{k}} < c_{hk}, q_{h\hat{k}} < q_{hk}.$$

By Propositions 18 and 19, $h\hat{k}$ is cost-effective relative to hk if and only if the expression in square brackets in (33) is non-negative or the expression in square brackets in (34) is negative. Each of these results occurs if and only if $B_{h\hat{k}} \geq B_{hk}$, so that if $h\hat{k}$ does not strongly dominate hk, $h\hat{k}$ is also cost-effective relative to hk if and only if $B_{h\hat{k}} \geq B_{hk}$. In addition, $B_{h\hat{k}} = B_{hk}$ when $h\hat{k}$ does not strongly dominate hk if and only if

$$R = \frac{c_{h\hat{k}} - c_{hk}}{q_{h\hat{k}} - q_{hk}},$$

and in that case $h\hat{k}$ and hk are cost-effective relative to one another. The proof is now complete.

Proposition 23. Treatment $h\hat{k}$ is or can be declared absolutely cost-effective for the focal illness h if and only if

$$B_{h\hat{k}} = \max_m \{B_{hm}\}.$$

And if and only if

$$B_{h\hat{k}} = \max_m \{B_{hm}\} = B_{hk}$$

for one or more $hk \neq h\hat{k}$, $h\hat{k}$ can be declared absolutely cost-effective or not for the illness as the health care agency prefers.

Proof: If

$$B_{h\hat{k}} = \max_m \{B_{hm}\}$$

either $B_{h\hat{k}} > B_{hk}$ for all $\hat{k} \neq k$ or else $B_{h\hat{k}} = B_{hk}$ for some hk. If $B_{h\hat{k}} > B_{hk}$ for all hk $\neq$ h$\hat{k}$, treatment h$\hat{k}$ is cost-effective relative to every other treatment for h by Proposition 22, and it is therefore absolutely cost-effective for h. On the other hand, if

$$B_{h\hat{k}} = \max_m \{B_{hm}\} \text{ and } B_{h\hat{k}} = B_{hk}$$

for some hk, h$\hat{k}$ and hk are cost-effective relative to each other and to every other treatment for h. Hence they are each absolutely cost-effective for h.

Now assume h$\hat{k}$ is absolutely cost-effective for the focal illness. Then by Proposition 22 it must be that $B_{h\hat{k}} \geq B_{hk}$ for every hk $\neq$ h$\hat{k}$. Hence

$$B_{h\hat{k}} = \max_m \{B_{hm}\}$$

and if h$\hat{k}$ can be declared absolutely cost-effective or not for h, there must be at least one other treatment hk that is also absolutely cost-effective for h. Accordingly,

$$B_{hk} = \max_m \{B_{hm}\}$$

by Proposition 22 and there exists a B_{hk} such that $B_{h\hat{k}} = B_{hk'}$. These last two results establish the necessity of the proposition's assertions and the proof is complete.

Remark 23. Notice that $B_{h1} = Rq_{h1} - c_{h1} = 0$. Hence

$$\max_m \{B_{hm}\} \geq 0$$

The last proposition of the section adds nothing to Proposition 23 but it facilitates the comparison of the net benefits and GM single-treatment decision rules given in the next section.

Proposition 24. Suppose hk is not strongly dominated but that it is weakly dominated by hp and hm, and that $c_{hp} > c_{hk} > c_{hm}$ and $q_{hp} > q_{hk} >$

q_{hm}. Then either hp or hm is cost-effective relative to hk.

Proof: By parts (ii) and (iii) of Proposition 2,

$$\frac{c_{hk} - c_{hm}}{q_{hk} - q_{hm}} \geq \frac{c_{hp} - c_{hk}}{q_{hm} - q_{hk}}.$$

Now treatment hk is cost-effective relative to treatment hm or it is not. If it is not, hm is cost-effective relative to hk and the claim is trivially true. If hk is cost-effective relative to hm, by Proposition 22,

$$B_{hk} - B_{hm} = (q_{hk} - q_{hm}) \left[R - \frac{c_{hk} - c_{hm}}{q_{hk} - q_{hm}} \right] \geq 0,$$

and the difference in square brackets must therefore be non-negative. However, in that event,

$$B_{hp} - B_{hk} = (q_{hp} - q_{hk}) \left[R - \frac{c_{hp} - c_{hk}}{q_{hp} - q_{hk}} \right] \geq 0$$

as well, and as a consequence hp is cost-effective relative to hk by Proposition 22. Thus one of the two treatments hm or hp is always cost-effective relative to hk, and the proof is complete.

It follows from the proposition's claim and the claim of Proposition 23 that a weakly dominated treatment is either not absolutely cost-effective or can be declared not absolutely cost-effective for h. There always exists at least one other treatment that is cost-effective relative to it.

8.3 The Equivalence of the Net Benefits and GM Decision Rules for Absolute Cost-effectiveness

As shown in Chapter 7 the MO single-treatment decision rules for absolute cost-effectiveness are, except possibly when $C = C^t$ for some t, the same as the GM single-treatment rules when the cutoff point is R(C). This suggests, of course, that with the same proviso the net benefits and GM decision rules for absolute cost-effectiveness are also the same. Yet the rules do not appear to be alike. For one thing, at the outset of the GM CEA the rules require that all dominated treatments be removed from the new treatment set for h before $\hat{hk}$ is tested for absolute cost-effectiveness, and the net benefits rules do not. In addition, the GM tests entail comparisons of the ICE ratio $R_{\hat{hk}}$ with ICE ratios defined on the ordered pairs of other treatments in the new treatment set, whereas in Proposition 23 ICE ratios play no direct part in the tests of the absolute cost-effectiveness of $\hat{hk}$. At all events, the outward dissimilarities between the net benefits decision rules and those of a GM and MO health care agency suggest that the two sets of rules are not the same. But the differences are only superficial, and it is therefore instructive to compare the two sets of rules in some detail.

1. As in a single-treatment GM CEA the costs and health benefits of all treatments for the focal illness must first be calculated or otherwise obtained. If there are treatments that are extraordinarily expensive and/or produce very few health benefits, they might reasonably be dismissed at the outset of the CEA as not absolutely cost-effective.

2. All nonstrictly strongly dominated treatments are for purposes of the CEA identical to the treatments that dominate them, and they and their dominating treatments are combined. If $c_{\hat{hk}} = c_{hk}$ and $q_{\hat{hk}} = q_{hk}$ for one or more of the initial hk, $\hat{hk}$ is merged with the hk and the composite treatment is relabeled $\hat{hk}$. In the net benefits decision rules it is unnecessary to delete other dominated treatments from the set of treatments for illness h because the net benefit rules ignore them. However, it does no harm to remove all dominated treatments from the set because none of them will be found to be or declared absolutely cost-effective. That is, when all nonstrictly strongly treatments have been merged, every remaining strongly dominated treatment is therefore strictly dominated, and if hk is weakly dominated there always exists a dominating treatment that is cost-effective relative to it (Proposition 24). Thus as in a GM CEA, $\hat{hk}$ is not absolutely cost-effective if it is dominated. A GM CEA terminates immediately if $\hat{hk}$ is found to be dominated, but because the net benefits rules do not require that

dominated treatments be deleted, a net benefits CEA will not. However, the net benefit rules do not forbid the removal of all dominated treatments, and if $h\hat{k}$ is dominated it will not be judged absolutely cost-effective. In that case and as in a GM CEA, $h\hat{k}$ can immediately be removed from the new treatment set and the net benefits CEA terminates as well.

3. If $h\hat{k}$ is not dominated, the next step in a GM CEA is to order the new treatment set so that treatment costs and health benefits increase strictly in the treatment index. The ICE ratios defined on adjacent treatments in the ordered set are next computed, and they too increase strictly in the treatment index. No ordering of the new treatment set or computations of the R_{hk} are required in a net benefits CEA because the net benefits rules are the same for all such orderings and they do not necessitate the values of the R_{hk}. However, again it does no harm to assume that the new treatment set has been ordered as it would be for a GM CEA and that the R_{hk} have been computed.

4. As in a GM CEA the health care system's cutoff point R must be known or taken as a parameter of the analysis. The net benefits of each treatment $B_{hk} = Rq_{hk} - c_{hk}$ must be calculated.

5. The net benefits rules (Proposition 23) now state that $h\hat{k}$ is absolutely cost-effective for h if and only

$$B_{h\hat{k}} = \max_m \{B_{hm}\}$$

unless it happens that there is an hk such that

$$B_{h\hat{k}} = B_{hk} = \max_m \{B_{hm}\}.$$

If there is such an hk, $h\hat{k}$ can be declared absolutely cost-effective or not as the health care agency prefers. The analogous maximum ICE-ratio (GM) rules state that $h\hat{k}$ is absolutely cost-effective for h if and only if

$$R_{h\hat{k}} = \max_m \{R_{hm} < R(C)\}$$

unless it happens that $R_{h\hat{k}} = R(C)$ or $R_{h\hat{k}+1} = R(C)$, and in that case $h\hat{k}$ can be declared absolutely cost-effective or not as the health care agency prefers.

Consider the maximum net benefit rule and the GM maximum ICE-ratio rule, and assume that $R = R(C)$. If there is no $B_{hk} = B_{h\hat{k}}$, $h\hat{k}$ is absolutely cost-effective for h if and only if

$$B_{h\hat{k}} = \max_m \{B_{hm}\}.$$

But by the ordering of treatment costs, treatment health benefits, and the R_{hm}, it is also the case that

$$B_{h\hat{k}} - B_{hk} = (q_{h\hat{k}} - q_{hk}) \left[R(C) - \frac{c_{h\hat{k}} - c_{hk}}{q_{h\hat{k}} - q_{hk}} \right] > 0 \text{ for all } k < \hat{k}$$

and

$$B_{hk} - B_{h\hat{k}} = (q_{hk} - q_{h\hat{k}}) \left[R(C) - \frac{c_{hk} - c_{h\hat{k}}}{q_{hk} - q_{h\hat{k}}} \right] < 0 \text{ for all } k > \hat{k}.$$

Thus provided there is no $B_{hk} = B_{h\hat{k}}$,

$$R_{h\hat{k}} = \max_m \{R_{hm} < R(C)\}$$

if and only if

$$B_{h\hat{k}} = \max_m \{B_{hm}\}.$$

Thus if there is no $C = C^t$, the net benefit maximum net-benefits and maximum ICE-ratio decision rules give the same conclusion as to the absolute cost-effectiveness of $h\hat{k}$.

Now assume there is a B_{hk} such that

$$B_{h\hat{k}} = B_{hk} = \max_m \{B_{hm}\}.$$

Hence by the ordering of the treatment set for h

$$B_{h\hat{k}} - B_{hk} = (q_{h\hat{k}} - q_{hk}) \left[RC) - \frac{c_{h\hat{k}} - c_{hk}}{q_{h\hat{k}} - q_{hk}} \right] = 0$$

and

(35) $$R(C) = \frac{c_{h\hat{k}} - c_{hk}}{q_{h\hat{k}} - q_{hk}} \text{ if } \hat{k} > k$$

(36) $$R(C) = \frac{c_{hk} - c_{h\hat{k}}}{q_{hk} - q_{h\hat{k}}} \text{ if } \hat{k} < k.$$

Suppose $\hat{k} - 1 > k$. Then if

$$B_{hk} = \max_m \{B_{hm}\},$$

$$B_{h\hat{k}-1} - B_{hk} = (q_{h\hat{k}-1} - q_{hk}) \left[RC) - \frac{c_{h\hat{k}-1} - c_{hk}}{q_{h\hat{k}-1} - q_{hk}} \right] \leq 0,$$

so that by Lemma 2,

$$R(C) \leq \frac{c_{h\hat{k}-1} - c_{hk}}{q_{h\hat{k}-1} - q_{hk}} < \frac{c_{h\hat{k}} - c_{hk}}{q_{h\hat{k}} - q_{hk}}.$$

This result contradicts (35) and the contradiction proves that $k \geq \hat{k} - 1$. Now suppose $k > \hat{k} + 1$. In that case,

$$B_{hk} - B_{h\hat{k}+1} = (q_{hk} - q_{h\hat{k}+1}) \left[RC) - \frac{c_{hk} - c_{h\hat{k}+1}}{q_{hk} - q_{h\hat{k}+1}} \right] \geq 0,$$

and again by Lemma 2,

$$R(C) \geq \frac{c_{hk} - c_{h\hat{k}+1}}{q_{hk} - q_{h\hat{k}+1}} > \frac{c_{hk} - c_{h\hat{k}}}{q_{hk} - q_{h\hat{k}}}.$$

These inequalities contradict (36) and the contradiction proves that $k \leq \hat{k} + 1$.

The demonstration that $\hat{k} + 1 \geq k \geq \hat{k} - 1$ implies that $k = \hat{k} - 1$ or $k = \hat{k} + 1$, and as a consequence that

$$B_{h\hat{k}} = B_{hk} = \max_m \{B_{hm}\}$$

if and only if $R_{h\hat{k}} = R(C)$ or $R_{h\hat{k}+1} = R(C)$. Hence if $R = R(C)$, there is a $B_{hk} = B_{h\hat{k}}$, and $C \neq C^t$, the net benefits and ICE-ratio decision rules give the same conclusion of the absolute cost-effectiveness of $h\hat{k}$. Treatment $h\hat{k}$ can be declared absolutely cost-effective or not as the health care agency prefers.

The equivalence of the net benefits and ICE-ratio decision rules for absolute cost-effectiveness of new treatments can be illustrated by three numerical examples. The costs and health benefits of treatments used in the examples are shown in Tables 8.1, 8.2, and 8.3. The tables are replicas, respectively, of Tables 6.3, 6.5, and 6.21 in Chapter 6 except for the rightmost columns that display the net benefits of the treatments for the illnesses. In the first two examples the focal illness is illness 3 and in the third it is illness 2. The GM cutoff point in the examples in Chapter 6—there numbered Examples 1, 2, and 8—is $25,000 per unit of health benefits, and the same cutoff point is assumed in the three examples presented here. In the third example the focal illness is of the cutoff-point type, but in the first two examples it is not.

In Example 1 in Chapter 6 it is shown that the treatment costs and health benefits in Table 8.1 imply that the new treatment 3a is absolutely cost-effective for illness 3. That is, the ICE ratio

$$R_{3a} = 20,000 < \max_{m} \{R_{3m} < 25,000\},$$

and by the GM maximum ICE-ratio rule 3a is absolutely cost-effective for the illness. The net benefits decision rule of Proposition 23 states that 3a is or can be declared absolutely cost-effective if and only if

$$B_{3a} = \max_{m} \{B_{3m}\},$$

Table 8.1
Treatment Costs, Health Benefits, Incremental Cost-Effectiveness Ratios, and Net Benefits for the New Treatment 3a for Illness 3
R(C) = $25,000 Per Unit of Health Benefits

Treat-ment	Cost per Treatment in $ (c_{hk})	Net Benefits per Treatment (q_{hk})	ICE Ratio	Net Benefits ($Rq_{hk} - c_{hk}$)
31	0	0	--	25,000x0 – 0 = 0
32	250	0.1	2,500	25,000x(0.1) – 250 = 2,250
33	1,000	0.25	5,000	25,000x(0.25) – 1,000 = 5,250
3a	1,800	0.29	20,000	25,000x(0.29) – 1,800 = 5,450
34	2,200	0.3	60,000	25,000x(0.30) – 2,200 = 5,300

Table 8.2
Treatment Costs, Health Benefits, Incremental Cost-Effectiveness
Ratios, and Net Benefits for the New Treatment 3a for Illness 3
R(C) = $25,000 Per Unit of Health Benefits

Treat-ment	Cost per Treatment in $ (c_{hk})	Net Benefits per Treatment (q_{hk})	ICE Ratio	Net Benefits ($Rq_{hk} - c_{hk}$)
31	0	0	--	25,000x0 – 0 = 0
32	250	0.1	2,500	25,000x(0.1) – 250 = 2,250
33	1,000	0.25	5,000	25,000x(0.25) – 1,000 = 5,250
34	2,200	0.3	24,000	25,000x(0.30) – 2,200 = 5,300
3a	2,800	0.32	30,000	25,000x(0.32) – 2,800 = 5,200

and by inspection of the rightmost column of Table 8.1 it is the case that B_{3a} is strictly larger than the net benefits of every other treatment for illness 3. Therefore, the GM and net benefits decision rules both imply that 3a is absolutely cost-effective for illness 3.

In Example 2 in Chapter 6 it is shown that the new treatment 3a, now assumed to cost $2,800 and produce 0.32 units of health benefits, is not absolutely cost-effective for illness 3 because by the maximum ICE-ratio decision rule

$$R_{3a} > R_{34} = \max_{m} \{R_{3m} < 25,000\}.$$

The appropriate net benefits decision rule for assessing the absolute cost-effectiveness of 3a is the maximum net-benefits rule, and by inspection of

the rightmost column of Table 8.2 it is evident that

$$B_{3a} < \max_{m} \{B_{3m}\}.$$

Thus by the net benefits methodology treatment 3a is also not absolutely cost-effective for illness 3. Last of all, consider the data for illness 2 presented in Table 8.3. In Example 8 in Chapter 6 it is shown that 2a can be declared absolutely cost-effective or not for illness 2 by the $R_{h\hat{k}} = R(C)$ or $R_{h\hat{k}+1} = R(C)$ decision rule. That is,

$$\frac{C_{43} - C_{4a}}{q_{43} - q_{4a}} = R(\$12 \text{ million}) = \$25,000.$$

To obtain this conclusion, the GM decision rules first call for treatment 23, which is nonstrictly weakly dominated by treatments 22 and 2a, to be removed from the treatment set for the illness. But to apply the net

Table 8.3
Treatment Costs, Health Benefits, Incremental Cost-Effectiveness Ratios, and Net Benefits for the New Treatment 2a for Illness 2
R(C) = $25,000 Per Unit of Health Benefits

Treat-ment	Cost per Treatment in $ (C_{hk})	Net Benefits per Treatment (q_{hk})	ICE Ratio	Net Benefits ($Rq_{hk} - C_{hk}$)
21	0	0	--	25,000x0 – 0 = 0
22	8,000	1.0	8,000	25,000x(1.0) – 8,000 = 17,000
23	12,000	1.16	25,000	25,000x(1.16) – 12,000 = 17,000
2a	17,000	1.36	25,000	25,000x(1.36) – 17,000 = 17,000

benefits decision rule

$$B_{h\hat{k}} = B_{h\hat{k}-1} \ (\text{or} = B_{h\hat{k}+1}) = \max_{m} \{B_{hm}\},$$

it is not necessary to make the removal. The four treatments' net benefits shown in the rightmost column of Table 8.3 indicate that $B_{2a} = B_{22} = B_{23} = \$17,000$. Thus whether or not treatment 23 is first removed from the treatment set, $B_{2a} = B_{22}$, and the net benefits rule therefore implies that the health care agency can declare treatment 2a absolutely cost-effective or not as it prefers. The rule does not assert that the total quantity of health benefits is the same for each option, but it is safe to draw that inference because the statement is explicit in the GM ICE-ratio rule and it and the net benefits rule are substantively equivalent.

The net benefits of any treatment hk, $Rq_{hk} - c_{hk}$, has no obvious or intrinsic meaning as a physical construct, and a health care agency has no rational cause for seeking to produce more than fewer net health benefits for the health wellbeing of its community. Rather, the value of the net benefits variable lies in its applicability to the decision rules of single-treatment CEA. It has been shown in this chapter that such decision rules exist for net benefits and that, except in a way that is of negligible empirical importance—that $C = C^t$—they give the same conclusions as the ICE-ratio decision rules of the GM and MO health care agency models. Hence the net benefits rules can be used in place of the ICE-ratio rules when the health care agency is taken to be either a global maximizer or a myopic optimizer, and they have certain operational advantages over the ICE-ratio rules. They do not require that dominated treatments be removed from the new treatment set, and the new treatment set need not be ordered so that they can be applied. This alone would seem sufficient to justify their use, but as was said at the beginning of the chapter, their principal attractive feature is their adaptability for testing the cost-effectiveness of new treatments statistically. The possibilities for devising statistical tests for that purpose are examined in the next chapter.

References

Stinnett AA, Mullahy J. Net health benefits: a new framework for the analysis of uncertainty in cost-effectiveness analysis. Medical Decision Making 1998; 18: S68-S80.

9 Probabilistic Methods of Single-Treatment Cost-Effectiveness Analysis

9.1 Introduction

Probabilistic methods are a relatively recent innovation in single-treatment CEA. The first kinds of single-treatment CEAs were performed deterministically, and the deterministic approach is still commonly employed. The approach consists first of defining a model of the treatment or treatments at issue. The models used in the CEA literature are variously called decision-tree, decision analytic, or Markov models. A treatment can be a simple one-procedure intervention such as an optometric examination for glasses (although even that can have several subsidiary procedures and outcomes if it includes screening for glaucoma and other optical problems), or it may be complex. For example, the diagnosis of a malignancy can consist of a number and series of tests, and patients may be given any one or more of these tests depending on the conclusiveness of the evidence obtained from the previous test or examination. In general, there are also four basic outcomes of a diagnostic treatment: false positive, false negative, correct positive, and correct negative, and except for the last of the four, each of them can have secondary outcomes of its own with further medical or surgical consequences.

In the course of designing a CEA, the components and structures of treatments are ordinarily set out by the organization for which the CEA is intended or by physician or other provider participants in the analysis who are familiar with the treatments' structures. When a particular treatment is sufficiently complicated, its procedures and their outcomes are often represented diagramatically as a branching process or tree (hence the name "decision-tree model"). A patient can be directed, guided, or instructed through a sequence of procedures depicted as pathways through the various branches of a tree, the trunk of which is the starting point of the treatment, perhaps the patient's presentation to a provider. In Markov terminology the procedures that the patient may undergo and outcomes she may experience are defined as states of being, and a patient undergoes treatment by proceeding in a special pathway from one state to another. To complete the treatment model for a CEA it is necessary to know the likelihoods—transition probabilities in Markov terminology—that a patient is directed, guided, or instructed to receive each particular procedure or experience its outcome following the outcome associated with a prior procedure or outcome. Depending on the availability of primary or secondary data, these probabilities can be estimated as the proportions of all patients who experience procedure or outcome A, then procedure or outcome B, A then C, B then C, and so on. If the suitable data are not available, the worst case option other than abandoning the CEA is to obtain estimates of the transition probabilities from an expert consultant or participant in the analysis.

The next step in this deterministic approach is to attach costs and health benefits to each procedure and outcome in the treatment model, and that can also be a challenging task. But once it is completed the analyst constructs the expected cost and health benefits of the treatment, and this done by weighting the costs and health benefits of each procedure or outcome—state—by the probabilities that they occur. The computations are routine and they yield point estimates of the treatment's cost and health benefits.

It was, of course, immediately realized by analysts that the point estimates of costs and health benefits for this kind of deterministic CEA are open to error and that the conclusions of the analyses are therefore potentially erroneous as well. Estimates of treatment costs are not necessarily perfectly correct, estimates of health benefits tend to vary with the instrument used to measure quality of life or with the conjectures of consultants, and the probabilities attached to treatment pathways can easily be misestimated as well. Accordingly, it quickly became standard practice in the empirical literature to subject the conclusions of single-treatment CEAs to sensitivity analyses.

These sensitivity analyses entailed varying the estimates of treatment costs, health benefits, pathway probabilities, or the parameters used to construct the estimates—and possibly also the assumed cutoff point—in order to evaluate the reliability of the CEA's conclusion. The conclusion was regarded less or more reliable to the extent that it did or did not change markedly in response to changes in the CEA's key parameters. Deterministic sensitivity analyses of this kind are still used in published CEAs, but they are only somewhat informative because they cannot be standardized and it is hard at best to make sense of or draw firm judgments of the CEA's result when three or more variables are changed simultaneously.

At least since the 1940s simulation methods have been employed in the engineering and applied sciences to evaluate the performance of especially complex physical systems. The use of Monte Carlo simulation to generate samples of data from decision-analytic models seems to have been proposed by cost-effectiveness analysts by the early 1990s, first as a device for conducting sensitivity analyses of the conclusions of CEAs. For a single-treatment CEA the method creates observations on the treatment model's costs, health benefits, or decision variables. The parameters of treatment costs and health benefits or the estimated costs and health benefits themselves are respecified as random variables and probability distributions are definied on them. The cost, health benefit, or decision variable data are then produced by computer software having random or probabilistic number generators, and a large number of these data can be created very quickly. Many desk-top software packages are marketed for Monte Carlo simulation and can be used to construct the sample data.

A second method for creating treatment cost, health benefit, and decision variable data is called bootstrapping, but it is usually applied to an original sample of observed data rather than to estimates derived from a decision-tree model. Samples of cost and health benefit data began to be collected for or applied to single-treatment CEAs by the 1990s, and when they were available these samples eliminated the need to construct decision-tree models and their cost and health benefit estimates based on secondary data and even conjectures. Bootstrapping is now a commonplace method in applied statistics for making many samples of data from an initial small one. Different bootstrapping procedures exist but the one most often proposed or used for single-treatment CEAs is known as nonparametric bootstrapping. It produces new samples of data by randomly choosing observations from the original sample with replacement. In particular, suppose the size of the initial sample is T. Then each subsequent sample is also of size T and each element of that sample is an observation from the initial sample selected with probability 1/T. Like Monte Carlo simulation, bootstrapping operations are performed with readily available computer software, and with it a large number of bootstrapped samples can also be quickly created.

Large samples of cost, health benefit, and decision variable data are increasingly employed in the empirical CEA literature for several reasons. As described in the next section, they are used to make descriptive estimates of the probability of the reliability of the CEAs' conclusions. But they are also helpful for parametric assessments of cost-effectiveness. In parametric applications of single-treatment CEA, normality is an advantageous property of decision variables because it permits the analyst to judge cost-effectiveness by means of conventional statistical methods. The Central Limit Theorem states that if a random variable has a bounded mean and variance, the probability distribution of its sample mean approaches the normal distribution asymptotically as the sample size becomes large. Hence if the decision variable in a CEA is the sample mean of a random variable having a bounded mean and variance, it is defensible to assume that this decision variable is approximately normally distributed in large samples. In addition, the variance of a sample mean approaches zero as the sample size becomes very large. Thus when the test for cost-effectiveness involves a particular value or interval of values of the decision variable, a large sample size gives confidence that the actual value of the decision variable is very little different from its sample mean estimate.

As this is written Monte Carlo simulation and bootstrapping are being increasingly used in published single-treatment CEAs, and it seems likely they will become regular features of the analyses as probabilistic methods are more widely accepted by researchers.

9.2   Estimating Confidence Intervals for Incremental Cost-Effectiveness Ratios

When empirical single-treatment CEAs were first performed they involved only two treatments, and two-treatment CEAs are still the most common type appearing in the literature. The convention is to say that a new or particular treatment $h\hat{k}$ is cost-effective if and only it is judged to be so in comparison with one other treatment hk according to an ICE-ratio-cutoff-point decision rule. More specifically, $h\hat{k}$ is customarily said to be cost-effective if and only if

$$R_{h\hat{k}k} = \frac{c_{h\hat{k}} - c_{hk}}{q_{h\hat{k}} - q_{hk}} < R,$$

where R is the health care agency's or the health care system's designated cutoff point. Probabilistic methods began to be applied in single-treatment CEAs as devices for conducted sensitivity analyses of the conclusions drawn from deterministic decision analytic treatment models. But when it became evident that large samples of data could be created from these models, it also became apparent that inferences could be made about the relationship between the estimate of $R_{h\hat{k}k}$ and R by examining the sample distributions of treatment costs and health benefits or, more directly, the distribution of the computed values of $R_{h\hat{k}k}$. The procedure generally gave easier to understand and more comprehensive

223

assessments of the reliability of the CEA's conclusion than did deterministic variations of treatment cost and health benefit parameters taken two or three at a time. However, it also became apparent that the CEA could be conducted directly with the use of either simulated sample data produced from decision analytic treatment models or bootstrapped data from an original sample of treatment costs and health benefits. Probabilistic assessments of two-treatment cost-effectiveness focussed first on estimating confidence intervals for the "true" value of $R_{h\hat{k}k}$, and the estimation of confidence intervals for $R_{h\hat{k}k}$ continues to draw the attention of researchers. To date a half dozen or more parametric and nonparametric methods for estimating these confidence intervals have been used or proposed. (For a representative selection of this literature see van Hout et al. [1994], Gardiner et al. [1995], Chaudhary and Stearns [1996], Willan and O'Brien [1996], Laska et al. [1997], Polsky et al. [1997], Tambour and Zethraeus [1998], Briggs et al. [1999], Campbell and Torgerson [1999], Heitjan et al. [1999], Glick et al. [2001], Wang and Zhao [2008], Gray et al. [2010]).

The simplest of the nonparametric methods consists of defining the "true" value of $R_{h\hat{k}k}$ as the mean of the probability distribution of the ICE ratio $R_{h\hat{k}k}$ and estimating it as the mean $\bar{R}_{h\hat{k}k}$ of the sample distribution of the $R_{h\hat{k}k}$. A confidence interval for the "true" $R_{h\hat{k}k}$ is then constructed by choosing a distance L such that the interval $\bar{R}_{h\hat{k}k} \pm L$ contains some pre-set percentage of all of the values of $R_{h\hat{k}k}$ computed from the observed $c_{h\hat{k}}$, $q_{h\hat{k}}$, c_{hk}, and q_{hk}. To set the interval's confidence interval at, say $(1-\alpha)\%$, the distance L is increased or reduced until the interval contains $(1-\alpha)\%$ of the computed $R_{h\hat{k}k}$. The usual parametric method for estimating the confidence interval is the textbook method. It also consists of constructing the interval $\bar{R}_{h\hat{k}k} \pm L$ but with the assumption that the sample mean of the distribution of $R_{h\hat{k}k}$ is normally distributed. The distance L for a pre-set α is then the product of the standard error of sample mean of the $R_{h\hat{k}k}$ and a number of standard deviations of the standard normal distribution determined by the probability α.

Although confidence interval estimation has played a large part in the evolution of probabilistic single-treatment CEA, its methods are now known to be unsustainable for at least three reasons. First of all, the probability that $h\hat{k}$ is "cost-effective" cannot be established by the single decision rule.

$$R_{h\hat{k}k} = \frac{c_{h\hat{k}} - c_{hk}}{q_{h\hat{k}} - q_{hk}} < R$$

because the decision rule is incorrect if $h\hat{k}$ is strongly dominated by hk. In that case either $R_{h\hat{k}k}$ is not defined or $R_{h\hat{k}k} < 0 < R$, and $h\hat{k}$ is therefore not cost-effective relative to hk. In addition, the rule is incorrect if $c_{h\hat{k}} < c_{hk}$, $q_{h\hat{k}} < q_{hk}$, and $R_{h\hat{k}k} < R$, since then

$$R_{h\hat{k}k} = \frac{c_{h\hat{k}} - c_{hk}}{q_{h\hat{k}} - q_{hk}} = \frac{c_{hk} - c_{h\hat{k}}}{q_{hk} - q_{h\hat{k}}} < R,$$

and by the rule hk, not $h\hat{k}$, is cost-effective. Indeed, under this last set of conditions on treatment costs, health benefits, and $R_{h\hat{k}k}$, $h\hat{k}$ is cost-effective if and only if $R_{h\hat{k}k} > 0$. Obviously, the anomalies can be managed by deleting sample observations such that hk strictly strongly dominates $h\hat{k}$ and that $c_{h\hat{k}} < c_{hk}$, $q_{h\hat{k}} < q_{hk}$, and $R_{h\hat{k}k} < R$. But when the deletions are made, an estimate of the probability that $h\hat{k}$ is cost-effective using only the maximum ICE-ratio rule is not unconditional. The estimate is conditional on the events that hk does not strongly dominate $h\hat{k}$ and that it is not true that $c_{h\hat{k}} < c_{hk}$, $q_{h\hat{k}} < q_{hk}$, and $R_{h\hat{k}k} < R$. Hence estimating the unconditional probability that $h\hat{k}$ is relatively cost-effective requires a somewhat more complicated procedure than merely estimating, if the estimate is justifiable, the conditional probability that

$$R_{h\hat{k}k} = \frac{c_{h\hat{k}} - c_{hk}}{q_{h\hat{k}} - q_{hk}} < R$$

given the deletion of data that cause the rule to be invalid.

The second problem with parametric confidence interval estimates of the "true" $R_{h\hat{k}k}$ is that it is hard to see how they bear on the question of whether $R_{h\hat{k}k}$ is smaller or larger than R. By supposition the ICE-ratio-cutoff-point rule $h\hat{k}$ is cost-effective if the "true" $R_{h\hat{k}k}$ is any point in the interval (0, R) or (0, R] depending on how the rule defines the right endpoint of the interval. But having an estimate of the confidence interval $\overline{R}_{h\hat{k}k} \pm L$ gives very little information about whether (0, R) or (0, R] contains $R_{h\hat{k}k}$. It could be claimed that if $R > \overline{R}_{h\hat{k}k} + L$ it is very likely that $h\hat{k}$ is cost-effective, and that if if $R < \overline{R}_{h\hat{k}k} - L$ it is very likely that $h\hat{k}$ is not cost-effective, but assigning exact probabilities to these events from the use of confidence interval estimates is questionable at best.

The third problem with confidence interval estimation of (or testing for) the "true" value of $R_{h\hat{k}k}$ is the dubious validity of the fundamental statistical assumptions on which the estimates (or statistical tests, if they are undertaken) are made. Up to this point the assumptions have been taken as supportable, but that is not necessarily the case. To begin with, unless the ICE ratio $R_{h\hat{k}k}$ is defined so as to exclude events such that $q_{h\hat{k}} = q_{hk}$ it cannot be assumed that it is normally distributed. If it is permitted that $q_{h\hat{k}} = q_{hk}$, $R_{h\hat{k}k}$ is unbounded, and a normal random variable cannot be unbounded. But even if $R_{h\hat{k}k}$ is defined so that $q_{h\hat{k}} \neq q_{hk}$, the claim that it or its sample mean is normally distributed is not defensible.

When treatment costs and health benefits are normally distributed, so are the differences $c_{h\hat{k}} - c_{hk}$ and $q_{h\hat{k}} - q_{hk}$, and therefore the ratio $R_{h\hat{k}k}$ is Cauchy distributed. The mean and variance of the Cauchy distribution are undefined—unbounded—and as a consequence the "true" value of $R_{h\hat{k}k}$ does not exist when it is defined as the mean of the sampling distribution of $R_{h\hat{k}k}$. Unless $q_{h\hat{k}} = q_{hk}$, a sample mean of observations on a Cauchy-distributed random variable can always be computed, but it cannot be argued persuasively that an observed sample mean is asymptotically normally distributed because the Central Limit Theorem's claim holds only for random variables having bounded means and variances. If treatment costs and health benefits are thought to be normally distributed, the premise that the mean of the distribution of an ICE ratio exists and that a meaningful confidence interval can be estimated for it is simply false.

It can, of course, be said that treatment costs and health benefits are not or are not necessarily normally distributed—they are, for example, always non-negative—but the Cauchy problem remains. Any claim that there exists a mean of the $R_{h\hat{k}k}$ and that a confidence interval can estimated for it requires more than the argument that treatment costs and health benefits are not necessarily normally distributed. If costs and health benefits are assumed to have special non-normal sample distributions, the sample distribution of R_{hk} must be derived and shown to be one having a bounded mean and variance. And this burden of showing the sample distribution of $R_{h\hat{k}k}$ to be tractable falls on the proponent of confidence-interval estimation, not on the user of its purported implications. Without a convincing proof and supporting evidence—and even if the other problems with the ICE-ratio decision rule could be resolved—the ICE-ratio-confidence-interval approach for decision-making in probabilistic CEA must be regarded as untenable.

There are descriptive and nonparametric methods that can be used for assessing cost-effectiveness with ICE ratios in two-way comparisons of treatments, but they can also be applied with net benefits decision variables, and without the defects of an incorrect decision rule and the questionable validity of confidence interval estimation.

9.3 Descriptive Methods of Probabilistic Cost-Effectiveness Analysis Using Net benefits Variables

The use of net benefits variables for probabilistic single-treatment CEA has two important advantages over the use of ICE ratios. The first is that the decision that $h\hat{k}$ is either relatively or absolute cost-effective can be made simply with a single variable. It is unnecessary to test separately that $h\hat{k}$ is or is not dominated; it is unnecessary to apply a second rule for anomalous events such that $c_{h\hat{k}} < c_{hk}$, $q_{h\hat{k}} < q_{hk}$, and $R_{h\hat{k}} \leq R$; and it is unnecessary to censor the samples of treatment costs and health benefits to exclude these events that give incorrect conclusions to the maximum ICE-ratio decision rule. By Proposition 22 $h\hat{k}$ is cost-effective or can be declared cost-effective relative to hk if and only if $B_{h\hat{k}} \geq B_{hk}$, and by Proposition 23 $h\hat{k}$ is or can be declared absolutely cost-effective for illness h if and only if

$$B_{h\hat{k}} = \max_{m} \{B_{hm}\}.$$

As was remarked in Chapter 8, the second methodological advantage of net benefits variables is their linearity in treatment costs and health benefits. Since $B_{hk} = Rq_{hk} - c_{hk}$, it follows that B_{hk} is normally distributed if if q_{hk} and c_{hk} are normally distributed and R is a constant. But even if it cannot be assumed that both q_{hk} and c_{hk} are normally distributed, it can be assumed that the means and variances of their distributions are bounded and hence by the Central Limit Theorem that their sample means are approximately normal in large samples. Thus whether $\bar{B}_{h\hat{k}}$ is defined as the sample mean of the observed $B_{h\hat{k}}$ or as

$$\bar{B}_{h\hat{k}} = R\bar{q}_{h\hat{k}} - \bar{c}_{h\hat{k}},$$

where $\bar{c}_{h\hat{k}}$ and $\bar{q}_{h\hat{k}}$ are the sample means of treatment costs and health benefits, it can reasonably assumed that $\bar{B}_{h\hat{k}}$ is approximately normally distributed in large samples.

There does, however, arise a methodological problem in translating the deterministic decision rules of Proposition 23 into probabilistic decision rules. In particular, the assertion that $h\hat{k}$ is cost-effective or can be declared cost-effective relative to hk if and only if $B_{h\hat{k}} \geq B_{hk}$, applies only to a single pair $B_{h\hat{k}}$ and B_{hk} of observations on net benefits variables. When there are many observations on the $B_{h\hat{k}}$ and B_{hk} it can ordinarily be anticipated that that there will be pairs for which $B_{h\hat{k}} \geq B_{hk}$ but also other pairs for which $B_{h\hat{k}} < B_{hk}$. Then some kind of probabilistic rule must be devised for deciding the issue of whether $B_{h\hat{k}}$ should be judged larger than or at least as large on balance as B_{hk}, and there is no unique way of specifying such a rule.

Essentially, two strategies are available for sample data. The first is to assess the probability that $B_{h\hat{k}} \geq B_{hk}$. The other is to determine whether the central tendency of the distribution of $B_{h\hat{k}}$ is at least as large as the central tendency of the distribution of B_{hk}, where central tendency is defined as the mean or median of the sample distribution. It seems fair to say that at present most analysts favor the probability strategy, but others have argued for comparisons of means or medians on grounds that $B_{h\hat{k}}$ should be judged cost-effective if and only if it is demonstrably "larger" than B_{hk} and not merely because it is "probably" larger. And, of course, there is no way to assure that the two analytic strategies always give the same conclusions. Nothing precludes the possibility that the estimated probability that $B_{h\hat{k}} \geq B_{hk}$ is positive and even statistically significant while at the same time and on account of a small number of observations in which B_{hk} is much larger than $B_{h\hat{k}}$, the sample mean of the $B_{h\hat{k}}$ is significantly smaller than the sample mean of the B_{hk}. Analysts may hope that this kind of conflict never arises, but if it does there is no logical way to resolve it. The analyst can only report her results, state that the CEA's conclusion is ambivalent, and leave the health care agency or other user to decide on what kind of action, if any, it will take in response.

The decision rules most often proposed and used in the recent cost-effectiveness literature center on the probability that $B_{h\hat{k}} \geq B_{hk}$ or that

$$B_{h\hat{k}} = \max_{m} \{B_{hm}\}.$$

The most popular of these approaches to decide the relative cost-effectiveness of $h\hat{k}$ employs a device called a *cost-effectiveness acceptance curve* (CEAC). A CEAC graphically displays the estimated probability that a new (or any) treatment $h\hat{k}$ is cost-effective relative to a comparator treatment for the same illness, and it is expressed as a function of the cutoff-point point R.

Two methods, one descriptive the other parametric, have been used or proposed in the CEA literature for estimating CEACs. The descriptive method (e.g., Fenwick et al. [2001]) consists of creating large samples of the costs and health benefits of treatments $h\hat{k}$ and a comparator treatment hk, choosing a cutoff point R, and then constructing large samples of $B_{h\hat{k}}$ and B_{hk} from the cost and health benefit data. The observations on the $B_{h\hat{k}}$ and B_{hk} are paired, and the probability that $B_{h\hat{k}}$ is cost-effective relative to B_{hk} is estimated as the proportion of all sample pairs in which $B_{h\hat{k}} \geq B_{hk}$ or $B_{h\hat{k}} > B_{hk}$ depending on how the analyst formulates the decision rule of Proposition 22. The procedure is repeated several or perhaps many times for different values of the cutoff point R, and its results are displayed graphically with values of R measured on the horizontal axis and values of the estimated probability of relative cost-effectiveness measured as points on the vertical axis. The point estimates are then connected by drawn lines or arcs, and the totality of the connected lines or arcs is the CEAC. The CEAC is now understood to display the estimated probability that $h\hat{k}$ is cost-effective relative to hk as a function of R.

These estimates are, of course, nonrigorous, and that fact appears to have induced some analysts to suggest a second parametric method of constructing CEACs, the basic premise of which is that incremental net benefits $B_{h\hat{k}k} = B_{h\hat{k}} - B_{hk}$ is normally distributed with density function $f(b|R)$. Then

$$\Pr[B_{h\hat{k}} \geq B_{hk}|R] = \Pr[B_{h\hat{k}k} \geq 0|R] = \int_{0}^{\infty} f(b \mid R)db ,$$

and the probability is estimated from tables or with software after the parameters of the density function have been estimated from sample data (e.g., Laska et al. [2002], Nixon et al. [nd]). To date the parametric method has not been widely used for estimating CEACs.

In whatever way a CEAC is estimated, it is left to the agency to choose the relevant cutoff point and decide the relative cost-effectiveness of a new treatment. The CEAC methodology is now used in empirical CEAs, but has also drawn criticisms the two most serious of which are that it gives an incorrect rule for judging cost-effectiveness and that it ignores the risk of error (e.g., Groot Koerkamp et al. [2007], Jakubczyk and Kaminski [2010]). The first criticism concerns the probabilistic meaning of "larger than" discussed at the beginning of the section. It holds that the goal of CEA is to choose treatments that produce the largest net benefits, not those that simply have high probabilities of producing more net benefits than other treatments. It is contended that a treatment should be judged cost-effective relative to a comparator if and only if it produces a larger expected net benefit than the comparator. The second criticism asserts that whether or not a CEA using the CEAC methodology indicates that a new treatment is (relatively) cost-effective, there remains a positive probability that the conclusion is wrong. Hence the CEAC methodology is said to have no mechanisms for helping the health care agency manage the risk of acting on false conclusions.

The first of the two criticisms is not supportable. It is true that showing $\Pr[B_{h\hat{k}} > B_{hk}]$ to be, say, significantly positive is not the only plausible way of concluding that $h\hat{k}$ is cost-effective relative to hk. But it is not true that $h\hat{k}$ should be judged relatively cost-effective only if the difference $E(B_{h\hat{k}}) - E(B_{hk})$ or median$(B_{h\hat{k}}) - $median$(B_{hk})$ is positive and large. Proposition 22 states that $h\hat{k}$ is cost-effective relative to hk if $B_{h\hat{k}} > B_{hk}$. The difference $B_{h\hat{k}} - B_{hk}$ may be large or small but the conclusion is the same. It is not the case that $h\hat{k}$ becomes "more" cost-effective relative to hk as the differences $B_{h\hat{k}} - B_{hk}$, $E(B_{h\hat{k}}) - E(B_{hk})$, or median$(B_{h\hat{k}}) - $median$(B_{hk})$ become larger. Moreover, it is not true that a rational utilitarian health care agency seeks more than fewer net benefits. The agency seeks more than fewer *health benefits*, and there is obviously no fixed relation between a quantity of health benefits and a quantity of net health or monetary benefits. The strongest form of the criticism of the CEAC decision rule must be that its implications are not logically unique. If a CEAC indicates that $h\hat{k}$ is relatively cost-effective but it also happens that the estimate of $E(B_{h\hat{k}}) - E(B_{hk}) < 0$ at some small significance level, the CEA's user would be justifiably reluctant to accept the CEAC's conclusion.

The second criticism is supportable. Like all descriptive statistical methods the CEAC approach does not attach probabilities to its findings, and setting a level of trust that can be placed on those findings is the task of the health care agency or other user. Standard statistical methods are available for evaluating the uncertainty of the estimated probabilities, but if risk is defined to include both uncertainty and the sizes of gains and losses due to fortuitous gains and losses due to adverse errors, more sophisticated decision-theoretic frameworks must be used.

Although it has long been understood by many analysts that relative cost-effectiveness is not sufficient reason for a health care agency to provide or sanction treatments for patients, few sampling methods have been devised for judging absolute cost-effectiveness. With one exception the methods that have appeared in the CEA literature are *ad hoc* or idiosyncratic, and they have not been widely adopted for empirical studies. The exception is a construction of net benefits called a *cost-effectiveness acceptability frontier* (CEAF). Given the cutoff point R the sample distribution of net benefits B_{hk} can be assumed to have a mean or expected value, say $E(B_{hk}|R)$, and when there are K treatments for illness h and K such expected values, it can be assumed there exists a largest of the expected values,

$$B(R) = \max_{m} \{E(B_{hm}|R)\}.$$

Then B(R) is the CEAF. That is, B(R) is the largest of all of the expected B_{hk} expressed as a function of the cutoff point R. Because the deterministic decision rule of Proposition 23 states that $h\hat{k}$ is absolutely cost-effective if

$$B_{h\hat{k}} = \max_{m} \{B_{hm}\},$$

it is natural to recast the rule in probabilistic form so that $h\hat{k}$ is absolutely cost-effective if

$$E(B_{h\hat{k}}) = B(R).$$

The expectations of the B_{hk} can be estimated parametrically (Laska et al. [2002]), but they are usually calculated descriptively from sample data (e.g., Barton et al. [2008]). Let there be a set of K treatments hk for illness h and assume that for each treatment hk a sample of size T_{hk} of the costs and health benefits has been collected or created. For each one of some set of values of the cutoff point R, compute T_{hk} values of B_{hk}. Denote these sample values by $b_{hk}^t(R)$, t = 1, 2, ..., T_{hk}. Next let $f_{hk}^t(R)$ be the relative frequency of $b_{hk}^t(R)$. The estimated expected value of B_{hk} given R is

$$\text{est. } E(B_{hk}|R) = \sum_{t=1}^{T_{hk}} f_{hk}^t(R) b_{hk}^t(R)$$

for all k > 1, $E(B_{h1}|R) = 0$, and

$$\text{est. } B(R) = \max_m \{\text{est. } E(B_{hk}|R)\}.$$

Then $h\hat{k}$ is said to be absolutely cost-effective for h at the cutoff point R if and only if

$$\text{est. } E(B_{h\hat{k}}|R) = \text{est. } B(R).$$

A number of point estimates of B(R) is often made, the points are displayed graphically, and, as is done with CEACs, the points are connected with lines or arcs so as to give a continuous function. This function of R is the CEAF. By comparing est. $E(B_{h\hat{k}}|R)$ = est. B(R) judgments of the absolute cost-effectiveness of $h\hat{k}$ can then be estimated for any value of R in the diagram.

Because the CEAF and its decision rule and the CEAC and its decision rule are both constructed and applied descriptively, some of the criticisms that have been made of the CEAC method can also be made of the CEAF method. The estimates used to decide absolute cost-effectiveness in the CEAF procedure and those used to decide relative cost-effectiveness in the CEAC procedure are both point estimates. Hence the decisions that $h\hat{k}$ is absolutely or relatively cost-effective are also essentially point estimates. They can vary from sample to sample of treatment costs and health benefits, and the CEAF and CEA procedures have no mechanisms for assessing their reliability and trustworthiness. Otherwise, analysts favoring the definition that "larger" in the net benefits decision theory should be taken as "most likely larger" and not "larger in magnitude" can argue that $E(B_{h\hat{k}}|R) = B(R)$ does not unambiguously make $h\hat{k}$ absolutely cost-effective. However, because the theory lacks established definitions of "larger than" and "largest", there are no logical ways of resolving the issue.

9.4 Statistical Tests for Absolute Cost-Effectiveness Using Net Benefits Variables

Although it would seem natural in a single-treatment CEA to test the cost-effectiveness of $h\hat{k}$ statistically, statistical tests have not yet been commonly used by analysts. There could be many reasons why this is so. No single statistical test for judging cost-effectiveness is completely defensible, and however the difference between $B_{h\hat{k}}$ and one other B_{hk} is defined, many different tests are available for deciding whether the difference is statistically significant. To apply one particular criterion of relative cost-effectiveness and one particular statistical test using that criterion could easily draw criticism, justifiable or not, that the analyst has failed to prove his case. As already mentioned, the issue of the risk of incorrect decisions has also sometimes been raised in discussions of probabilistic CEA. While this risk is not always precisely defined, it presumably refers to health care agencies' losses of health benefits, money resources, or both when they accept and act on the incorrect conclusions of CEAs. The probabilities of error are attached to the inferences of ordinary Neyman-Pearson statistical tests, but the tests are not designed and not equipped to evaluate error risks defined as losses of health benefits or money resources. This may also partly explain why Neyman-Pearson tests seem not to be used or proposed for single-treatment CEAs, and it is possible that other decision-theoretic procedures such as those incorporating loss functions or gaming against nature may eventually be preferred by health care agencies and health policy administrators concerned with risk. Then not last, any test for absolute cost-effectiveness using net benefits variables is a test that determines whether $B_{h\hat{k}}$ is larger than all the other B_{hk}. Statisticians have developed tests that are appropriate for deciding absolute cost-effectiveness, but the most rigorous approach to the question requires a derivation of the distribution of the largest member of a set of random variables, and that problem is as yet incompletely solved in the statistics literature. The statistical tests that do exist for assessing absolute cost-effectiveness are not without limitations, but until statistical theory becomes more advanced they deserve to be considered the most suitable instruments for conducting single-treatment CEAs.

It is not the intention in this book to propose exact procedures for carrying out CEAs—designing the problem, defining and compiling treatment costs and health benefits, and the like. But the net benefits variable was created and has become used for probabilistic CEA, and for that reason it is appropriate to consider a few of the possibilities for testing absolute cost-effectiveness statistically with the net benefits variable. It has been said in the preceding chapters that a treatment's absolute cost-effectiveness should be the *sine qua non* for an agency's decision to provide or sanction a treatment for its patients. Even so, there can be circumstances in which demonstrating the relative cost-effectiveness of $h\hat{k}$ also demonstrates its absolute cost-effectiveness. For example, if the illness was not previously cared for, $h\hat{k}$ is absolutely cost-effective if it is cost-effective relative to the no-action treatment. Or if hk is the only current treatment for the illness that is not minimally effective or prohibitively expensive, it is reasonable to think that $h\hat{k}$ is absolutely cost-effective if it is cost-effective relative to hk. Readers acquainted with elementary statistics will know that there are many tests for deciding whether or not $\Pr[B_{h\hat{k}} > B_{hk}]$ is significantly positive and for deciding whether or not the sample mean or median of the observed $B_{h\hat{k}}$ is larger than the sample mean or median of the observed B_{hk}. These tests will therefore not be discussed here.

Sign Tests for absolute cost-effectiveness.   Sign tests for absolute cost-effectiveness extend the CEAC methodology. Assume it is agreed that $h\hat{k}$ is absolutely cost-effective if and only if the probability

$$\Pr[B_{h\hat{k}} = \max_m \{B_{hm}\}]$$

is large. Assume there are K active treatments for illness h including $h\hat{k}$ and that a large sample of size T of the costs and health benefits of each treatment including $h\hat{k}$ has been created. For each of the K treatments compute the observed set of net benefits and let each such set be denoted $\{b_{hk}^1, b_{hk}^2, ..., b_{hk}^t, ..., b_{hk}^T\}$. Sort the data into a new set of T samples each of which contains exactly one observation on each b_{hk}^t. Now add the number 0 to each such set to denote the net benefit of the no-action treatment $B_{h1} = 0$. Then each of the T samples is of size K+1, it has the form $\{0, b_{h2}^t, ..., b_{hk}^t, ..., b_{hK}^t, b_{h\hat{k}}^t\}$, and each observed value of $B_{h\hat{k}}$ is matched with a complete set of the observed values of the other B_{hk} including $B_{h1} = 0$. This kind of matching is appropriate if each set of costs and health benefits data is observed, produced, or created simultaneously for all K active treatments. It is also appropriate if there is reason for believing that the conditions that generate each particular set $\{b_{h1}^t, b_{h2}^t, ..., b_{hk}^t, ..., b_{hK}^t, b_{h\hat{k}}^t\}$ are the same but may vary from set to set. But it is appropriate even if the b_{hk}^t are not inherently matched. If they are randomly generated, any set of the b_{hk}^t for $k \neq \hat{k}$ can be matched meaningfully with $b_{h\hat{k}}^t$.

If $B_{h\hat{k}}$ is larger than the other B_{hk}, the proportion of the T samples in which $b_{h\hat{k}}^t$ is the largest of the b_{hk}^t should itself be large, and a test for the absolute cost-effectiveness of $h\hat{k}$ can therefore be framed as a test on the value of a sample proportion. The larger is the proportion of all T samples in which $b_{h\hat{k}}^t$ is the largest element, the more likely is it that

$$B_{h\hat{k}} = \max_m \{B_{hm}\}.$$

To state the statistical test formally, make it that $h\hat{k}$ is absolutely cost-effective for illness h if and only if

$$\Pr[B_{h\hat{k}} = \max_m \{B_{hm}\}] = P_{h\hat{k}} > P^*,$$

where P* is a threshold probability selected by the user of the CEA. A health care agency might not settle for knowing only that the probability is significantly positive that $B_{h\hat{k}}$ is the largest of the B_{hk}. This probability can, of course, be significantly positive and still be very small. Hence depending on the agency's risk preference P* can be chosen as any value ≥ 0 and < 1, but the more risk averse the agency is the larger P* is likely to be. (Notice that if $B_{h\hat{k}}$ is as large as but no larger than the other B_{hk} and 0, the true probability that $b_{h\hat{k}}$ is a member of the largest T of the observed b_{hk} is $1/(K+1)$. It would therefore be reasonable to choose P* no smaller than $1/(K+1)$). To use the Neyman-Pearson framework, the test for the absolute cost-effectiveness of $h\hat{k}$ is then a test of the null and alternative hypotheses

$$H_o: P_{h\hat{k}} \leq P^* \ (h\hat{k} \text{ is not absolutely cost-effective})$$

$$H_1: P_{h\hat{k}} > P^* \ (h\hat{k} \text{ is absolutely cost-effective}).$$

This formulation of the hypotheses presumes the user of the CEA is risk averse and will not decide that $h\hat{k}$ is absolutely cost-effective unless the empirical evidence favoring that conclusion is sufficiently convincing. If the user is a risk taker the hypotheses can be reversed. Notice that for test purposes H_o is equivalent to the hypothesis $P_{h\hat{k}} = P^*$.

The statistical test is now a simple one that is described in elementary textbooks. Define the Bernoulli variable

$$x^t = \begin{cases} 1 \text{ if } b_{h\hat{k}}^t \geq \max_m \{0, \text{ all } b_{hm}^t, | \, m = 1, 2, ..., K\} \\ 0 \text{ otherwise} \end{cases}$$

for $t = 1, 2, ..., T$. Then x^t is distributed binomially with

$$Pr[x^t = 1] = P_{h\hat{k}} = Pr[B_{h\hat{k}} = \max_m \{B_{hm}\}].$$

The estimator of $P_{h\hat{k}}$ is

$$p_{h\hat{k}} = \sum_{t=1}^{T} x^t / T,$$

and if the number of samples T is large, it can be assumed that $p_{h\hat{k}}$ is normally distributed. Supposing the null hypothesis is true, the test statistic is

$$d_{h\hat{k}} = \frac{P_{h\hat{k}} - P^*}{\sqrt{P^*(1-P^*)/T}},$$

and provided T is large, $d_{h\hat{k}}$ is normally distributed with mean 0 and standard error 1. It is then decided that $h\hat{k}$ is absolutely cost-effective (H_o is rejected) at the α significance level if and only if the estimate of $p_{h\hat{k}}$ is "large"—if and only if the estimate of $d_{h\hat{k}} > z_\alpha$, where $Pr[Z > z_\alpha] = \alpha$ and Z is a standard normal random variable.

Inasmuch as health care agencies and other users of the CEA may have different preferences toward the risk of false positive conclusions regarding the absolute cost-effectiveness of $h\hat{k}$, it would usually be desirable for the analyst to report the test result for some number of different values of P^* and α. If R is regarded as an unknown or uncertain parameter, the result should also be reported for some appropriate set of values of R. Again, the more averse agencies and other users of the CEA are to the risk of a false conclusion that $h\hat{k}$ is absolutely cost-effective, the larger are the values of P^* and the smaller are the values of the significance level α they will prefer.

If the analyst believes it is not defensible to match each $b_{h\hat{k}}$ with a any particular set of the other b_{hk}, another simple sign test is also available. Again merge the T samples of the b_{hk} and add a "sample" of T zeros to represent the b_{h1}. The total sample is of size $(K+1) \times T$. Order the b_{hk} from smallest to largest and consider the subsample of the T largest of these b_{hk}. Call the subsample LargeB. If there are tied values of the b_{hk} so that the subsample cannot be chosen uniquely, choose the smallest of the groups of tied values and remove at random as many of the tied values as are necessary to make the size of LargeB exactly T. Then define the Bernoulli variable

$$x^t = \begin{cases} 1 \text{ if } b_{h\hat{k}}^t \text{ is in LargeB} \\ 0 \text{ otherwise} \end{cases}$$

for $t = 1, 2, ..., T$, and

238

$$Pr[x^t = 1] = P_{h\hat{k}} = Pr[B_{h\hat{k}} = \max_m \{B_{hm}\}].$$

The argument here is that if and only $B_{h\hat{k}} \geq B_{hk}$ and there are T observations on each set of the observed net benefits, then many or all of the largest T observations should be observations on $B_{h\hat{k}}$. Thus the larger is the proportion of the $b_{h\hat{k}}$ among the members of LargeB, the more likely it is that $B_{h\hat{k}} = \max_m \{B_{hm}\}$. As before, the estimator of $P_{h\hat{k}}$ is

$$P_{h\hat{k}} = \sum_{t=1}^{T} x^t /T.$$

The null and hypotheses are the same as those of the matched sample test. The decision statistic is the same and the test is performed in the same way as well.

Parametric tests. Assume now it is agreed that $h\hat{k}$ is absolutely cost-effective if and only if the mean of the distribution of $B_{h\hat{k}}$ is at least as large as) the mean of the distribution of every other B_{hk} including $B_{h1} = 0$. It can, of course, be reasonably assumed that the means and variances of the distributions of all of the B_{hk} exist.

Let $\beta_{h\hat{k}}$ be the mean of the distribution of the $B_{h\hat{k}}$ and let β_{hk} be the mean of the distribution of the net benefit B_{hk}, k = 1, 2,..., K. Then estimators of $\beta_{h\hat{k}}$ and the β_{hk} are the sample means of observed net benefits $\overline{b}_{h\hat{k}}$ and $\overline{b}_{hk}$ (with $\overline{b}_{h1}$ = 0), and the simplest test for deciding whether $\beta_{h\hat{k}} > \beta_{hk}$ is to determine separately for each pair of sample means whether $\overline{b}_{h\hat{k}}$ is significantly larger than $\overline{b}_{hk}$. Treatment $h\hat{k}$ can be judged absolutely cost-effective if and only if $\overline{b}_{h\hat{k}}$ is significantly larger than every $\overline{b}_{hk}$ including $\overline{b}_{h1}$ = 0. If it is believed that the costs and health benefits of $h\hat{k}$ are in some way matched with the costs and health benefits of the other hk, the appropriate tests are two-sample paired means tests. Otherwise, the tests are two independent-sample means tests. (Notice that sample medians can be used in polace of sample means.) Two-sample means (and median) tests are described in most elementary statistics tests and need not be discussed here.

The problem with this kind of strategy is that the overall level of significance of the K tests—that probability that one or more of them gives a false conclusion that $\beta_{h\hat{k}} > \beta_{hk}$—cannot easily be determined. However, a well-known theorem variously named the Bonferroni procedure, correction, or adjustment states that the joint significance level of K independent tests is no greater than the sum of the K individual significance levels (e.g., Glantz [2000], Kleinbaum et al. [2013], Nolan and Heinzen [2012], Rosner [2010]). Thus if the two-sample strategy is undertaken, it should be decided that $h\hat{k}$ is absolutely if and only if $\bar{b}_{h\hat{k}} > \bar{b}_{hk}$ significantly at the α_k level for every treatment hk, k = 1, 2,..., K, and the joint significance level of the tests is then no larger than $\sum \alpha_k$. If the individual sample sizes T are large enough, it may be possible to constrain $\sum \alpha_k$ to a pre-set level. Otherwise, the significance levels of the individual tests might be set at α/K or in some other defensible way so that $\sum \alpha_k$ equals a pre-set joint significance level α. The test results should be reported for some appropriate set of values of $\sum \alpha_k$ and R.

A test procedure more explicitly suited for comparing the means of net benefits in a single-treatment CEA is one-way analysis of variance (ANOVA) and a *post hoc* test for its results. Like the other procedures discussed in this section, the methods of one-way ANOVA are well known and can be performed with readily available statistical software (e.g., Dean and Voss [1999], Doncaster and Davey [2007], Gamst et al. [2008]). Here the ANOVA is a test for significant differences among the sample means of net benefits, $\bar{b}_{h\hat{k}}$, $\bar{b}_{h1}$, $\bar{b}_{h2}$,..., $\bar{b}_{hK}$. The samples of net benefits need not be the same size but it is useful for *post hoc* tests of ANOVA's results if they are. If the sample sizes are the same, it should be assumed that a faux sample of zeros of the given size (for the no-action treatment h1) is added to the K samples of observations on the net benefits of active treatments. (Nothing in the ANOVA procedure precludes it; for example, it could happen that all observations on an activity actually are zeros.) The test's null hypothesis is that the true means—the means of the distributions of the observed net benefits—are equal. Its alternative hypothesis is that at least one of these means is different from the others.

By the deterministic Proposition 23 $h\hat{k}$ can arbitrarily be declared absolutely cost-effective or not if $B_{h\hat{k}} = B_{hk}$ for another hk, but a test result indicating that the sample means of $B_{h\hat{k}}$ and B_{hk} are significantly different does not, of course, imply that $h\hat{k}$ can be said to be absolutely cost-effective. Applying the deterministic decision rule in this uncertain case is obviously likely to produce false conclusions. For practical purposes the appropriate rule is that $h\hat{k}$ is absolutely cost-effective if and only if $\bar{b}_{h\hat{k}}$ is significantly positive and significantly larger than the sample means of the net benefits of all other active treatments. Because opinions may differ among users of the CEA regarding the correct value of the cutoff point and the test's significance level, it would be useful to perform the ANOVA for some preset number of different values of the cutoff point and significance level. The finding that there are or are no significant differences among mean net benefits will ordinarily vary with the assumed cutoff point and significance level. As it is with sensitivity analyses of deterministic CEAs' results, conclusions of the ANOVA that change with changes in the cutoff point and significance level might reasonably be taken as evidence that $h\hat{k}$ is not, or is not clearly, absolutely cost-effective.

The ANOVA's result may be difficult to interpret. For example, if there are no significant differences among the sample means of the B_{hk}, it implies that $c_{hk}/q_{hk} = R$ for every k (since $B_{1k} = 0 = B_{hk} = Rq_{hk} - c_{hk}$). And it also implies that every treatment including the no-action treatment is cost-effective relative to every other treatment for h. On the other hand, if there are significant differences among the sample means, it can be possible to conjecture a conclusion of the absolute cost-effectiveness of $h\hat{k}$. If, say, $\bar{b}_{h\hat{k}}$ is the smallest of the sample means it would be reasonable to infer that $h\hat{k}$ is not absolutely cost-effective for h, and if $\bar{b}_{h\hat{k}}$ is the largest of the sample means it would be reasonable to think that $h\hat{k}$ is or can be declared absolutely cost-effective for h. But even in these cases it is advisable that the analyst make his decision more precisely by conducting a *post hoc* test on the differences between $\bar{b}_{h\hat{k}}$ and the other sample means of net benefits.

In the past half century a dozen or more sujitable *post hoc* ANOVA tests have been devised by statisticians, the best known and most often used of which are named after their authors—the Fischer, Scheffè, and Tukey tests. Although it is not the most conservative of the three tests, the Tukey test is the most often recommended because it is the most powerful of the three (the most likely to imply that the means of the K distributions are different when, in fact, they are different). All three tests can be performed with standard statistical software such as SPSS and SAS. For a pre-set significance level α each of the tests constructs a single interval, say $D(\alpha)$, derived from the mean square error of the ANOVA and an ordinate of the t- or F-distribution such that the differences $\bar{b}_{hm} - \bar{b}_{hk}$ are all significantly positive at the α level if $\bar{b}_{hm} - \bar{b}_{hk} > D(\alpha)$ for every k = 1, 2,..., K. Thus it can be concluded that $h\hat{k}$ is absolutely cost-effective for h at the α significance level if and only if $\bar{b}_{h\hat{k}} - \bar{b}_{hk} > D(\alpha)$ for every k = 1, 2,..., K.

The most suitable *post hoc* ANOVA test is, however, known as Dunnett's or the Dunnett test. The test was created to determine whether the mean response of a particular group subjects or objects is numerically larger or smaller than the each of the mean responses of a particular group of other subjects or objects. In the context of single-treatment CEA the response of the first group is the net benefit of treatment $h\hat{k}$ and the responses of the comparator groups are the net benefits of the other hk. The test has not been used in single-treatment CEAs but it would appear to be especially appropriate for the problem of deciding absolute cost-effectiveness. The test is described in statistics texts (e.g., Bechhofer et al. [1995], Miller [1998], Dean and Voss [1999], Quinn and Keough [2002], Field [2009]) and it is contained in statistical software packages like SPSS and SAS.

A comparison of the desirable and undesirable features of statistical tests for absolute cost-effectiveness goes well beyond the purposes of this book, and the tests described here by no means exhaust the number and variety of those that could be used in single-treatment CEAs. Still, statistical tests should be regarded as preferable to the kinds of descriptive methods currently used in the CEA literature to assess cost-effectiveness. It is not that descriptive methods are of no value, but statistical tests are as informative as descriptive methods and, unlike descriptive methods, they give users of CEAs probabilistic measures of the reliability of the information they convey.

No attempt has been made in this chapter to suggest an ideal or perfectly acceptable statistical test or group of tests for absolute cost-effectiveness. In all likelihood no such test or group of tests exists. There can be legitimate disagreements about how the deterministic criterion stating that $h\hat{k}$ is absolutely cost-effective if

$$B_{h\hat{k}} = \max_m \{B_{hk}\}$$

should be formulated when there two or more values of both $B_{h\hat{k}}$ and each of the B_{hk}. And even if agreement should emerge on how this reformulation should be made, selecting a most convincing, most trustworthy, most powerful, or most acceptable test becomes a task for statistical theorists.

Nevertheless, based on what is now known of the principles of single-treatment CEA, there can be little doubt that the net benefits theory should be the preferred framework for decision-making in probabilistic single-treatment CEAs. The net benefits decision rule for absolute cost-effectiveness is both simpler to use than the treatment dominance and ICE-ratio decision rules and also much easier and more defensible to apply when there are multiple sample values of treatment costs and net benefits. This is not to say, however, that the treatment dominance and ICE-ratio decision rules are irrelevant. By itself, neither the net benefit $B_{h\hat{k}}$ nor its relations with other net benefits have any intrinsic theoretical or ethical content. It is the theoretical and ethical content of the GM and MO health care agency models that make the net benefits decision rules of Proposition 23 meaningful. The net benefit rules should be preferred for conducting either deterministic or probabilistic single-treatment CEAs, but these rules are empty and unintelligible without the substance given them by the GM and MO health care agency models.

References

Barton GR, Briggs AH, Fenwick EAL. Optimal cost-effectiveness decisions: the role of the cost-effectiveness acceptability curve (CEAC), the cost-effectiveness acceptability frontier (CEAF) and the expected value of perfection information (EVPI). Value in Health 2008; 11: 886-897.

Bechhofer RE, Santner TJ, Goldsman DM. Design and Analysis of Experiments for Statistical Selection, Screening, and Multiple Comparisons. New York: Wiley, 1995.

Briggs AH, Mooney CZ, Wonderling DE. Constructing confidence intervals for cost-effectiveness ratios: an evaluation of parametric and non-parametric techniques using Monte Carlo simulation. Statistics in Medicine 1999; 18: 3245-3262.

Campbell MK, Torgerson DJ. Bootstrapping: estimating confidence intervals for cost-effectiveness ratios. Quarterly Journal of Medicine 1999; 92: 177-182

Chaudhary MA, Stearns SC. Estimating confidence intervals for cost-effectiveness ratios: an example from a randomized trial. Statistics in Medicine 1996; 15: 1447-1458.

Dean AM, Voss D. Design and Analysis of Experiments. New York: Springer, 1999.

Gardiner J, Hogan A, Holmes-Rovner M, Rovner D, Griffith L, Kupersmith J. Confidence intervals for cost-effectiveness ratios. Medical Decision Making 1995; 15: 254-263.

Doncaster CP, Davey AJH. Analysis of Variance and Covariance: How to Choose and Construct Models for the Life Sciences. New York: Cambridge University Press, 2007.

Fenwick E, Claxton K, Sculpher M. Representing uncertainty: the role of cost-effectiveness acceptance curves. Health Economics 2001; 10: 779-787.

Field A. Discovering Statistics Using SPSS. Thousand Oaks, CA: Sage, 2009.

Gamst G, Meyers LS, Guarino AJ. Analysis of Variance Designs: A

Conception and Computational Approach with SPSS and SAS. New York: Cambridge University Press, 2008.

Glantz SA. Applied Regression and Analysis of Variance (2nd ed). New York: McGraw-Hill, 2000.

Glick HA, Briggs AH, Polsky D. Quantifying stochastic uncertainty and presenting results of cost-effectiveness analyses. Expert Review of Pharmacoeconomics and Outcomes Research 2001; 1: 25-36.

Gray AM, Clarke PM, Wolstenholme J, Wordsworth S. Applied Methods of Cost-Effectiveness Analysis in Healthcare. New York: Oxford University Press, 2010.

Groot Koerkamp B, Hunink MGM, Stijnen T, Hannitt JK, Kuntz KM, Weinstein MC. Limitations of acceptability curves for presenting uncertainty in cost-effectiveness analysis. Medical Decision Making 2007; 27: 101-111.

Heitjan DF, Moskowitz AJ, Whang W. Problems with interval estimates of the incremental cost-effectiveness ratio. Medical Decision Making 1999;19: 9-15.

Jakubczyk M, Kaminski B. Cost-effectiveness acceptability curves—caveats quantified. Health Economics 2010; 19: 955-963.

Kleinbaum DG, Kupper LL, Nizam A, Rosenberg ES. Applied Regression Analysis and Other Multivariate Methods. Boston: Cengage Learning, 2013.

Laska EM, Meisner M, Siegel C. Statistical inference for cost-effectiveness ratios. Health Economics 1997; 6: 229-242.

Laska EM, Meisner M, Siegel C, Wanderling J. Statistical determination of cost-effectiveness frontier based on net health benefits. Health Economics 2002; 11: 249-264.

Miller RG. Beyond ANOVA: Basics of Applied Statistics. Boca Raton, FL: Chapman and Hall, 1998.

Nixon RM, Wonderling D., Grieve R. How to estimate cost-effectiveness acceptability curves, confidence ellipses and incremental net benefits alongside randomized controlled trials. MRC Biostatistics Unit, Institute of Public Health, Cambridge UK, n.d.

Nolan S, Heinzen T. Statistics for the Behavioral Sciences. New York: Worth Publishers, 2012.

Polsky D, Glick HA, Willke R, Schulman K. Confidence intervals for cost-effectiveness ratios: a comparison of four methods. Health Economics 1997; 6: 243-252.

Quinn GP, Keough MJ. Experimental Design for Biologists. New York: Cambridge University Press, 2002.

Rosner B. Fundamentals of Biostatistics. Boston: Brooks/Cole Cengage Learning, 2010.

Tambour M, Zethraeus N. Bootstrap confidence intervals for cost-effectiveness ratios: some simulation results 1998; 7: 143-147.

Van Hout BA, Al MJ, Gordon GS, Rutten FF. Costs, effects, and c/e ratios alongside a clinical trial. Health Economics 1994; 3: 309-319.

Wang H, Zhao H. A study of confidence intervals for incremental cost-effectiveness ratios. Biometric Journal 2008; 50: 505-514.

www.ingramcontent.com/pod-product-compliance
Lightning Source LLC
Chambersburg PA
CBHW051449170526
45166CB00001B/168